Guide Her Home

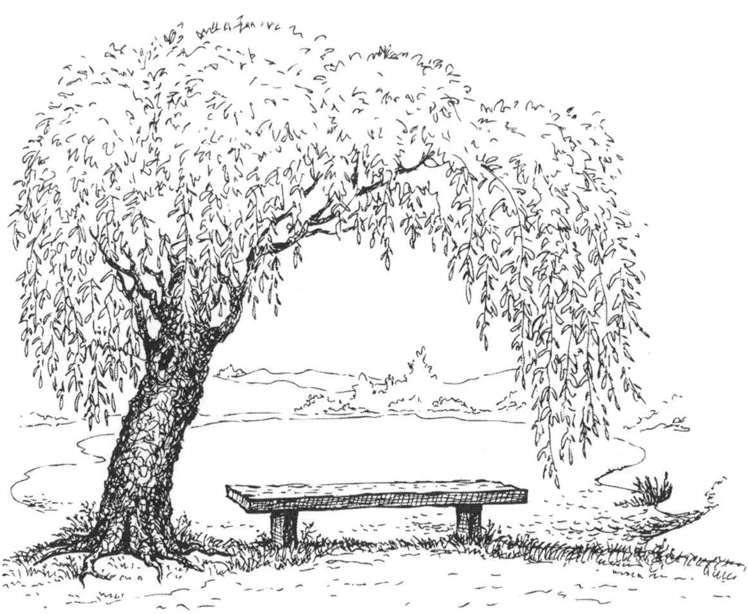

Guide Her Home

A Year of Hope After a Child's Tragedy

Jolene Lavine

MAKE IT SHINE CREATIONS
Vancouver, Washington

Permission requests should be sent to:
GHH Requests
C/O Jolene Lavine
15640 NE Fourth Plain Boulevard, Ste. 106 #47
Vancouver, WA 98682

No information contained in this book should be considered professional advice or services to the individual reader.

Cover images: Dreamstime.com (Mother Daughter Kiss ©Sarah Nicholl, Angel Winged ©Rolffimages, Willow Tree By The Lake ©Maryna Kriuchenko)

Cover design: Diane M. Papadakis, DMP Publishing, www.DMPpublishing.com

Interior design: Williams Writing, Editing & Design, www.williamswriting.com

ISBN-10: 0-9904371-4-0
ISBN-13: 978-0-9904371-4-7

For everyone who told me
I needed to write this book
and
those who believed I could do it,
starting with one drunken night
when I was nineteen years old.

CONTENTS

VARIATION UN

VARIATION DEUX

CODA

AUTHOR'S NOTE

If you have been around our family at all in the years following Jessica's accident, there may come a time when you are reading this book... very possibly from the very first page... when you think to yourself, *That's not how it happened.*

You may be right. Although this story is based on actual events, some details have been moved or combined to help with the flow of the story. Also, some people have been combined into one character while the names and identifying details of others have been changed to protect their privacy.

Please forgive me if something isn't painted in the light of your memory. There are three sides to every story: yours, mine, and the truth.

As I say in the disclaimer on the Viva La Jessica! Facebook Community page, "The information contained within this story is from a mother's perspective. While these pages are public, I am not a trained medical doctor, nurse, physiatrist, physical therapist, occupational therapist, speech therapist, cognitive specialist, neurosurgeon, neurologist, internist, gastroenterologist, pediatrician or psychologist."

I *am* a mother who is fiercely dedicated to her children. That can be blinding sometimes.

This is what I remember.

This is my perspective.

Thank you for taking this journey with me.

Jolene Lavine

ENTRÉE

I wish I could show you, when you are lonely or in darkness, the astonishing light of your own being.

Hafiz

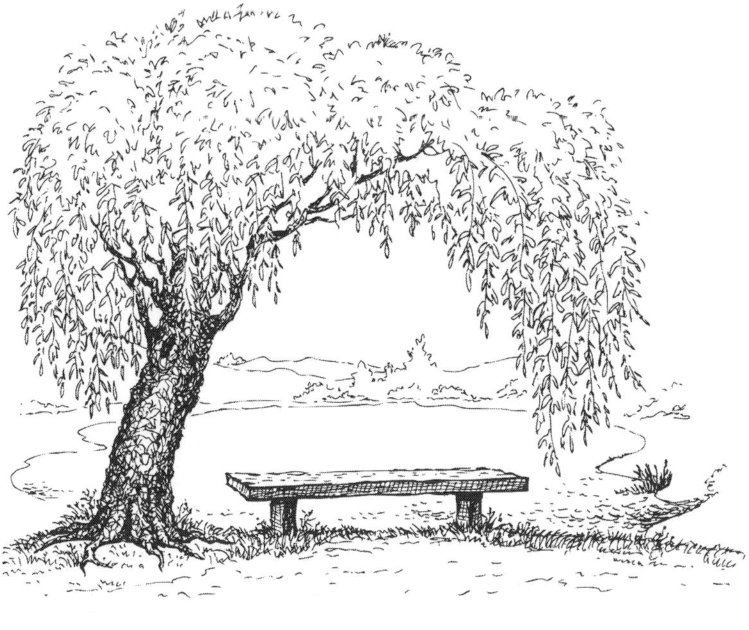

PROLOGUE

Before we were born, Jessica and I sat around in the Great Unknown, comparing notes and talking about the charts we were writing for our next go-round on this teeny blue-green planet. We compared our past lessons, talked about how easy they had been so far, and sighed about how we couldn't think of any more challenges.

"We need a real doozy," one of us (me, I'd guess) said. "Something to teach me patience, the true patience I've never quite found. The kind of abiding faith that knows whatever will be, will be as it should be. Deep and permanent and unwavering commitment would be a great thing to learn, too. And maybe... I dunno... I think I still have a little problem with trust. Especially trusting myself. I need one big, huge event that can help me with all of these. You have any ideas?"

Jessica said, "Well, I think I need to find confidence in myself no matter what the circumstance. I need to find inner strength. And I definitely need to learn I am powerful, that I can and should direct my own life. I need my next lesson to show me I am strong and do not need to follow or lead. I just need to be me. So I figure I could have this accident. No biggie, you know. Just a critical, life-threatening accident. It shouldn't be something that's anyone's fault but something challenging enough to require me to find my inner resources. What I'm suggesting still sounds pretty easy, but it'll probably be harder than most other stuff. Hard enough to help me evolve further, anyway."

"That's a good idea," I mumbled, processing Jessica's suggestion. "Maybe I need something like that... nah, that wouldn't help me.

I know my own power. I learned that already. Gotta think. There has to be something."

"Well, it could be... I mean, if you don't have anything planned yet... the accident could happen when I'm just a kid, and you could be my mom. But only if you can't think of your own challenge, of course."

"Hey, that's good! That just might work. Are you sure? You really want me to be your mom?"

"Yeah! It'd be great. We've already been through so many past lives together; how hard could it be?"

CHAPTER ONE

Speaking Words of Wisdom

April 29, 2010

It starts like any other Thursday.

Well, not really. On Wednesday night, Jessica requested French toast for breakfast. While it is her favorite, at age ten she doesn't often request breakfast from me. Her typical morning routine includes making toaster waffles or pouring a bowl of cereal before school. "Mom" breakfasts are a weekend treat or saved for special occasions, so when she made that special request, I agreed.

I open my eyes to see her sweet face smiling at me.

"You said you'd make French toast."

"Good morning, girlfriend," I whisper, reaching out to touch her cheek. "I remember. Let me freshen up, and I'll be right there."

Crawling out of bed, I check the clock to confirm we really have enough time before we head out the door for school. I groan when the clock informs me it is plenty early for French toast. I could have slept in a bit longer.

"What?" Jesse mumbles from under the covers. I wave him away while heading to the bathroom, knowing he's already fallen asleep again. I don't want to make too much noise, as he is snuggled up with our two-year-old Jocelyn, who crawled into our bed again last night.

While I wash the sleep from my eyes and swish some mouthwash around, I mentally run through our family schedule. Then I head to the kitchen.

"Aw, thanks for your help, Baby Girl." I smooch the top of Jessica's head and grab the ingredients she has already pulled from the fridge and cupboards.

"You're welcome, Mom." She hops onto the counter to reach the plates in the cupboard.

"Are you excited about competition this weekend?"

"Of course I am. Can I still buy stuff at the book fair today?"

"Yes. Remind me to give you a check before we leave. I'll need to show you how to fill it out, too."

She nods and sets a plate on the counter before jumping down and running off to her room to get dressed and grab her backpack.

While her breakfast cooks on the griddle, I pull the Crock-Pot out of the cupboard.

"I found a new recipe for tonight," I tell Jess when she returns from her bedroom, dressed in blue jeans and her favorite purple T-shirt covered with peace signs, guitars, and funky designs. Her glasses are perched on her nose, and brown hair falls to her shoulders, framing her round face.

"What is it?" She climbs up on the barstool that sits on the opposite side of the kitchen counter and takes the plate I slide toward her, as well as the syrup.

"It's a Crock-Pot chicken made with both mushrooms and onions." Her eyes light up. Mushrooms and onions are Jessica's two favorite vegetables.

We chat for a moment, and I watch her add just the right amount of syrup to each slice of toast. She grins at me through most of the bites. I take one more moment to enjoy her smiling face before returning to my bedroom to change clothes for the drive to school.

Once Jocelyn and I return home, I assemble dinner in the slow cooker before taking a shower and figuring out how we will keep busy while Jesse is at work.

We occasionally go to playgroup or shop, but most of the time we stay home to clean, read books, or watch a video. I always worry about what time Jocelyn will go down for a nap. She is still at the age where she needs about three hours to maintain her good mood, and since I pick up Jessica at 2:20, I try to put Jocelyn down for a nap by 11:00.

Thursdays are a different story, because the elementary school has "early release" and all classes are let out at 1:05. Trying to get Jocelyn down for a nap early enough to meet this early deadline is an exercise in futility, so I simply plan on her falling asleep in the car as I drive Jessica to her horseback riding lesson, which is right after school.

This works out well, because the older and more mobile Jocelyn gets, the more restricted she is at the barn where Jessica's lessons are held. She is too small to be around the horse enclosures, because there is the possibility of her spooking the horses. While she snoozes in the car, I take advantage of the time to read or catch a quick nap, too.

Jocelyn is definitely tired as we pull away from the house to pick up Jessica. I keep my eye on the rearview mirror, watching her eyes grow heavier and heavier on the short drive. She is too excited to see her sister, though, and we reach the school without her dropping off completely.

She starts to get a little whiny until I point out that the kids are starting to walk out of the building and Jessica will be along shortly. She scans the crowd for her sister while playing with a blanket. As the kids begin to make their way down the small hill on which the school sits, I roll down my window and concentrate on keeping a smile on my face as Jessica and her classmates emerge with the other students. The open window allows me to hear Jessica talking to her friends, which gives me a sense of how her day went.

Fourth grade hasn't been easy for Jessica. My girl definitely takes after me. She wants to get along with everyone and doesn't understand the dynamics and motivations of other fourth-grade girls. Their ability to hurt others cruelly one day and smile to their faces the next causes her pain far too often. She handles it better than I did at her age, however. No matter how much she hurts, she keeps smiling and attempts to be the bigger person. I'm sure she doesn't always succeed. I'm sure fourth-grade drama leads her to give in to spiteful behavior, as well. But what I typically see is Jessica trying, again and again, to be a good friend. Sadly, her efforts are wasted on girls who don't know any better.

Girls like Livia.

Jessica and Livia have been best friends since we moved to Orangevale a year and a half ago. Of course, being in the fourth grade means the term *best friend* is a bit of a grey area. BFFs one day, enemies the next.

Early in the school year, Livia's mom and I had many discussions, because every time Livia would tell on Jessica, her mother would phone me. It's easy for me to get sucked into drama, especially when it comes to my children, so we adults would dissect the construct of the girls' conflict and assure one another that this is a Very. Serious. Matter. Discussions with the girls would follow and when the pattern repeated itself a few times, I finally woke up and realized what should have been obvious from the beginning: *This is normal fourth grade behavior.*

I realized Livia's mom and I were fueling the fire the girls had been building, so I told Jessica she needed to learn to deal with it. While I can be there to give her advice and support her if that advice fails, she needs to play this social game on her own.

I tried to give her an edge by having extensive discussions about friendship and forgiveness. We talked about how to be a good friend and what type of treatment to accept from other people. Apparently, I hadn't hit the right combination of advice, since Jessica would forgive Livia over and over again, and Livia, possibly guided by her mother, continued to treat Jessica poorly.

Jessica finds solace in the friendships she has had since preschool days and in visits with her cousins, who are close to her age. She keeps busy performing with her competition dance troop and being involved in Girl Scout activities, and any pain she's feeling evaporates the minute she saddles up. Still, the daily struggles with a girl who wants to hang out with her one minute and ditches her the next wears on her.

In turn, it wears on me.

Today, as I watch the kids from Jessica's class, I notice that Livia is walking down the path ahead of Jessica next to another girl. She periodically looks over her shoulder to be sure Jessica hasn't caught up with her.

My anger begins to rise, and petty thoughts about "other people's children" begin to emerge, but I catch myself, take a deep breath, and remember to smile as Jessica reaches the van and climbs in.

"Hi, baby. How was school?"

"Good." She flashes her cute smile and shoves her backpack and a plastic shopping bag onto the floor by her feet. After closing the van door, she turns to lean into the back seat. "Hi, Jocelyn." She grabs her little sister's feet, and Jocelyn smiles and giggles. Jessica chatters to her before straightening up and reaching for her seat belt.

As we pull out into traffic, I ask about her purchases at the book fair.

"Oh!" She grabs the shopping bag and reaches inside.

In an effort to allow Jessica to learn more about money, responsibility, and independence, I'd followed through on my promise to give her a check and had shown her how to fill it out. Of course, she had a spending limit, but she was so excited and proud to be able to make a grown-up purchase without Mom hanging around.

As she pulls out her treasures, I'm not surprised to see animal-related books tumble into her lap, including *Five True Dog Stories* and *Heroic Animals*.

"Is that all you were able to get?"

"Nope. I got these, too." She fishes a pencil and eraser out of the bag. "I also bought pencils for Livia and Hope."

My smile falters a little, but I try to keep my voice light. "Oh, yeah?"

"Yep." She returns her books to the bag and begins kicking off her sneakers in order to change into her riding boots. While her giving nature is one of the qualities I cherish, it is also the reason I am so frustrated by the love/hate relationship with her best friend. My daughter is thoughtful enough to buy her buddy a pencil at the book fair just two hours earlier, and the girl repays her by leaving the school so quickly that Jessica can't walk with her. I know Jessica isn't perfect, but I've seen the way Livia treats other kids, so my patience with this relationship is quickly eroding.

Today the conflict is too much, and I find it impossible to keep my mouth shut. "Honey, it was sweet of you to buy gifts for your friends, but you need to be careful about that in the future."

"Why?"

"You want to be aware that people might take advantage of you."

She leans back in her seat, looking at me, eager to understand what I am failing to say outright. Guiding her toward more rewarding relationships while not poisoning the well against a child she clearly is drawn to is my biggest challenge. I also know she needs to be a kid. I don't want to squash her giving nature, the sweet side of her that finds value in being generous with her friend, regardless of how that person treats her.

On this day, when I have watched Livia racing ahead to avoid Jessica, my protectiveness wins out, and I begin to explain it to her. "Some people will want to be your friend because of what you can do for them, like buying presents. That's called taking advantage of someone. I want you to be aware."

She doesn't respond immediately. Her boots lay forgotten on the floor as she stares out the window at the scenery passing by.

I shift in my seat and realize that I should have let her be a kid today. A glance in the rearview mirror confirms that Jocelyn is sleeping soundly, and I ask Jessica softly, "What are you thinking, babe?"

She's equally quiet in her response. "Just trying to figure out if that's what happened."

I sigh and focus on driving, trying to think of a way to fix this. When we turn onto the long road that will eventually lead to the barn, I grab her hand and squeeze hard. "I'm sorry, baby. I shouldn't have said anything. Buying gifts for Livia and Hope was very sweet, and I'm sorry to have taken that from you. If all we have to worry about is whether you should buy a fifty-cent pencil for a classmate, then we really are pretty lucky."

"What do you mean?"

"Well, honey, what do we talk about all the time? We talk about gratitude and appreciating everything we have. That doesn't mean just stuff but other parts of life, as well."

"Like how you always say to look on the bright side?"

"Yes. Like that. Our family is so blessed, honey. There are people who have to deal with problems much bigger than anything we have going on. They have to worry about a place to live or having enough food to eat. We are blessed not to have to worry about those issues. We are healthy; we have shelter, clothes, and food. We are able to help those less fortunate—"

"Like we do with Girl Scouts?" She is nodding along and cuts me off, her understanding of what I'm saying sinking in. We're clutching tight to one another's hands, our voices soft and cracking with emotion at times. Teaching my children to appreciate all we have is important to me. These are lessons I learned way too late in life. It touches me deeply when Jessica, at ten years old, shows that she understands and reflects the lesson back to me. Jessica's tender heart comes to her naturally, and conversations like this can leave us hugging and laughing at each other through our tears. Having an emotional conversation in the car is definitely challenging.

"Yes, like we do with Girl Scouts. We are able to spread the blessings we are fortunate enough to have. So if you want to spend fifty cents to buy your friend a pencil, you should. I'm sorry I made a big deal about it. I want you to be happy, and sometimes I go about that the wrong way."

Jessica squeezes my hand again. As we drive the winding road to the barn, we continue our conversation about how immense *Gratitude* can be. I confess to being overprotective and remind her of the beauty in the world and the beauty in our lives, mentioning all we have to be grateful for. Blessings that are more important than money.

As we pull into the driveway of the barn and our conversation begins to wind down, she gets serious again. "But, Mom, we do have to worry about health stuff. And money, too."

"Well, of course we do, honey. Everyone does. It's just a matter of how serious our worries are. What are you thinking of specifically?"

"Well, when Grandpa died and we had to pay for his funeral."

My breath escapes me as I pull around the outside arena and into a parking spot next to the main barn. I put the car in park but leave it running. The stillness of the car may wake Jocelyn and I want to finish the conversation with Jessica before she heads off to her lesson.

My dad passed a little over a year ago, on the day that we closed on the purchase of our first house. The hardest part was telling Jessica her grandpa was gone. In the emotional days that followed, it never occurred to me that she knew we contributed to his funeral expenses.

My dad had been called "the strongest man in the world." Although congestive heart failure slowly stole his strength as he got older, Jessica wasn't old enough to see that. To her, he always would be the strongest man in the world.

She loved the way he teased her when they fought over *his* chair, and I can still picture him carrying her on his shoulders on their way to the park. My favorite photo is of the two of them together; her smile is so perfect and sweet.

He was the only other person in the room when I sang my first song to her shortly after she was born ("You Gotta Be" by Des'Ree), and he nicknamed her *Rosie* because her cheeks were always so pink. That nickname has become one of her favorites.

I turn to her now and take both of her hands in mine. "Oh, honey." It's a struggle to keep my voice level. "I know it was so hard to lose Grandpa. I know you miss him, and we will love him forever and ever. But he was sick for a very long time. Even though it hurts when someone dies, it's a natural part of life that everyone has to deal with. I don't know what I would do if something ever happened to you or Jocelyn. I don't know what I would do."

Keeping my voice level has become a losing battle, and Jessica climbs over the center console to hug me tight, crying softly on my shoulder. We sit there for a minute, and then both of us take a deep breath. She falls back in her seat, wiping her eyes with her shirt.

"Okay, enough of this. Get your boots on. Go find Miss Becky." We laugh softly at ourselves and how emotional we are together. She keeps glancing at me for smiles, and I supply them eagerly, worried about having such a deep conversation when she's still so young. She smiles at me, finishes pulling on her boots, and hops out of the van. Before heading off to find her instructor, she leans back in to give me a quick kiss.

"I love you, Mom."

"I love you, too, Peanut Butter. So much."

My worry begins to evaporate as she grabs her helmet, closes the door, and skips off toward the big barn.

I sit and breathe for a minute before finally turning off the engine.

I pick up my phone and send Jesse a text: *Wow. I just had a huge conversation with Jessica.*

I then open the Facebook app to get caught up on my newsfeed.

Jesse replies to my text, but before I read his response, I update my own Facebook status: *I need to stop making such a damn big deal about things. Life is good. I need to let it be.*

Suddenly, I hear yelling.

CHAPTER TWO

Heaven Sent a Hurricane

I don't think too much of it, figuring people are yelling to one another across the property. Glancing in the rearview mirror, I see someone coming toward the van. I open the door and lean out.

Blonde, eyes wild, phone in her hand, she is motioning for me to follow her while speaking into the phone. "I don't know; I am not there right now." To me she says, "Come with me."

I look at Jocelyn, sleeping peacefully, and start to object. "I can't, my daughter..." I gesture toward the backseat.

"You need to come. Your daughter..."

I look at Jocelyn again as the realization crashes over me, and I'm running.

The phone. Her wild eyes. *It's panic.*

"What happened?" I yell at her as we run the two hundred feet to the pasture. I can't begin to imagine what compelled the woman to have me leave my young child alone in the car. All of the possible scenarios crash together in my mind, and my inner truck driver escapes. "Mother fucker, mother fucker, mother fucker, mother fucker."

I reach the gate to the pasture and stop for a split second to take in the scene.

She's on the ground.

I don't have time to process the look on Becky's face as she leans over Jessica before I'm doing a home-plate slide into the dirt.

So much blood. There is so much blood. What happened? What happened? What happened? What do I do? What do I do?

And that's when I hear it. Unmistakably loud and comforting. I may not believe in much, but I do believe in Angels, and they are descending upon us and encircling us with their wings. I allow the peace and calm they provide to fill me up, and I begin whispering to Jessica.

"You are exactly where you should be. Mother Earth is supporting you, sending her energy up to cradle you. Our Angels are here surrounding us, and Grandpa is here, honey, and you are going to be fine. You are going to be fine. You are going to be fine."

I take a deep breath and almost immediately regret it, as the smell from the nearby manure pile fills my nostrils. I take a moment to look at Becky and the blonde woman. "Where is the ambulance?" I ask calmly.

They are both frantic. "I don't know. We called them. They don't know where we are!"

"My phone is on the console between the two front seats in my car. Please bring it to me." I refocus my energy on my girl and repeat the mantra. "You are going to be fine."

So much blood. Her ear is split. She's sniffing. Why is she sniffing? She has blood in her nose. So much blood.

"You are going to be fine. Just breathe and rest in the Angels' wings, baby. Grandpa is here. He will protect you. You are right where you need to be, and you are going to be fine."

The blonde woman returns with my phone, and I dial 911. I try to keep my voice calm when the operator answers. "My daughter has been in an accident at her horse barn. The people here called but said you don't know where we are. We are directly on Natoma-Bidwell road. It is Masters Riding and Boarding."

"Where is your daughter now?"

"She's on the ground. We're afraid to move her. She was struck on the right side of the head. There is a lot of blood, and it looks like her right ear is split open."

"Is she breathing?"

Could it be possible for her not to be? Oh, what is going on?

"She is. She is trying to clear the blood out of her nose. There is a lot of blood. Do you know where we are?"

"We do. Help is on the way. They should be there any—"

I look up to see the ambulance pulling up the barn road. "They're here. Thank you."

I shove the phone in my pocket and struggle to ground myself, trying to comfort Jessica once more. "Help is here now, baby. I know you're scared. I know it hurts, but you are going to be fine. Just breathe. You are going to be fine. You are going to be fine. You are going to be fine."

I'm not sure how I got there, but all of a sudden I'm standing by the passenger door of the ambulance. The blonde woman is next to me, and one of the medics is telling me to stay calm. I glance at his nametag, which reads "J. Green," and raise my eyes to his face. "What do I do?" I ask him.

"Get in," he says. His tone implies it's a repeated order. He's holding the passenger door open.

"My purse. My purse is in the van."

Without another word, the blonde woman runs off again, and J. Green gently pushes me into the ambulance. As the blonde hands my purse through the window, I grab her arm. "Please stay with my other daughter. I will call my husband right now. Please stay with her."

She is nodding and looks no less panicked than she did when she summoned me just moments before.

The short bursts of the siren announce our departure, and I grab my seatbelt as we pull away from the pasture. I twist in my seat to see what they're doing to Jessica, but one of the two paramedics is blocking my view. I want to ask what's happening and how my daughter is doing, but I can hear them talking in rapid bursts as they pull instruments from their sterile packaging. They are trying, trying so hard, to get a response from Jessica. I don't want to interrupt their work, so I grab my phone from my pocket and call Jesse.

My inner trucker makes another appearance when his cell phone goes straight to voicemail. I hang up and dial his work line, pushing the numbers of his extension with shaking hands.

"D-5. This is Jesse."

"I need you to leave right now. Jessica was kicked by a horse at the barn. I had to leave Jocelyn at the barn. Go get her. I need you to leave right now. Right now! I don't care what you are doing. I need you to come. Now."

His response barely registers with me as I end the call and dial my best friend's work number. Thankfully, she answers on the first ring.

"This is Kari."

The ambulance is loud and shaking as we make our way through the rural roads to the freeway, just minutes away.

"It's me." I speak louder than necessary, hoping she can hear me over the ambulance noise. "Jessica was in an accident at the barn."

I grab the door bar as the ambulance speeds onto the freeway and ask the driver, "Where are we going?"

"Sutter Roseville. That's the closest trauma center."

I speak into the phone. "We are going to Sutter Roseville. Can you please come?"

"Yes, let me wrap things up. Don't worry, honey. I will be there as soon as I can."

I hang up the phone again, and my focus returns to the medics working on Jessica. Their pace is less rushed, and they begin to ask me questions.

"What is your daughter's full name?"

"Jessica Ember Margaux Lavine." *My fiery child of light.*

"Date of birth?"

"March 21, 2000." *First day of spring. Emergency C-section.*

"Is she allergic to any medications?"

"None that we know of."

She's never had more than a cold a day in her life. We haven't had cause to find out if she's allergic to medication.

I try to listen to the driver as he calls our arrival into the hospital but start to feel dizzy, so I study my phone, trying to determine who to call next. I locate the number for one of my fellow dance moms, Barb. I have no idea what will happen once we hit the hospital, and I want to ask if she will take Jocelyn until we know what's going on.

"We're almost there," the driver tells me gently. I put my phone in my pocket, loop my purse over my shoulder, and take a deep breath as we round the corner and the hospital comes into view. The last few moments of the drive take the longest, with the driver carefully making his way through the parking lot and reversing into the ambulance bay.

I get out and head to the rear of the ambulance. The doors pop open, and the medics jump out and begin to maneuver the gurney out of the rig. I try to check on Jessica, but the gurney is still half in and half out. My eyes are drawn to the ground, where one of Jessica's black cowboy boots has fallen. I quickly stoop down and snatch it up, clutching the boot to my chest. The medics finish pulling Jessica out of the ambulance, and I follow them into the emergency room.

As if being blocked by one of the magical forcefields that appear in the fantasy books Jessica loves to read, I stand frozen at the emergency room doors as the gurney disappears into an orange sea. Dozens of nurses and doctors are waiting for us. All of them in orange scrubs. They move into action, racing to save my daughter's life, and I shake off the hand of a hospital employee who is trying to lead me away.

"I need to take you to register," the employee tells me.

"I need to watch until she's gone." One of Jessica's favorite movies plays in my head now. "It's tradition."

Jessica's gurney disappears behind the curtain, and I face the older gentleman, eager to follow him and get more information on what to expect next. He leads me out of the emergency room and around the side of the hospital so we can enter the lobby.

I follow him to the registration desk and listen as he begins to explain to the woman behind the admitting desk why we're there. "This is... There's..." He stumbles over his words, not having a clue who I am or what has happened. I look at the woman he's addressing and feel a small sense of relief as a familiar face greets me.

"Stacey. It's Jessica. Jessica is in the emergency room." Stacey is the mother of a child who was in Jessica's third-grade class.

"Oh, my gosh. Okay, come here." She grabs a chart from the desk and leads me to the waiting area. "Just fill this out, and I'll be right back."

CHAPTER THREE

Did I Say That I Need You?

Stacey seats me at one of the couches in the waiting room and hands me a clipboard. I try to read the form, but the letters are a jumbled mess. After making a half-hearted attempt to fill in the obvious blanks, I give up, looking for anyone who might be able to help me.

A tall, thin man wearing a hospital tag approaches me, and I stand to address him. He holds out his hand to shake mine and motions to the chairs. "I'm Jim Williams, a chaplain here."

"Excuse me?" I'm standing again before my butt has a chance to hit the seat, frantically looking for a doctor, Jesse, Stacey, or anyone other than a chaplain, who I imagine can only be there to offer one kind of comfort. "Has something happened to Jessica?"

"No, Ms. . . ."

"Lavine." My eyes are glued to the doors through which I'm sure my girl will emerge, bandaged up but all smiles.

"Ms. Lavine, I'm sorry. Please." He motions to the chairs again. "I don't have any news, but I am here to help in any way I can. I'm here to support you."

I turn to face him, not quite trusting what he's saying. "Can you find out where Jessica is? I need to be with her. I can't stay here." I look toward the door again.

He stands now, following my gaze. "Let me see if I can get any information for you." He disappears, and a movement to my left catches my eye. Becky is coming through the lobby doors. She spots me and rushes over.

"How is she?"

"I'm trying to find out where she is. I need to be with her."

Becky puts one hand over her heart, and I grab her free hand. "What happened?" I ask. Then I wave the air between us, as if I can swat the question away. "Never mind. Not now."

Becky squeezes my hand, and I scan the area again, hoping to find someone who can lead us to my girl.

The chaplain walks toward us with a short brunette woman wearing glasses and carrying a stack of papers. She extends her hand and says, "Ms. Lavine? Come this way." I have no idea who she is or where she's taking me, but anything is better than this spacious, vaulted lobby with floor-to-ceiling windows. At any other time, I am sure I would be impressed by the space and the light. Right now, I feel lost and exposed.

Becky and I rush to follow the chaplain and the woman into a hallway. They stop in the middle of the corridor, and the woman explains. "In a moment, they will bring your daughter through these doors." She motions to the double doors to the right. "They will cut straight across to imaging, where they will perform a CT scan of her brain.

"Once they have the CT scan, they will go to that elevator at the end of the hall," she says, motioning behind her. "It will proceed straight to the surgery floor. They will be moving fast. If there is room in the elevator, you may join them. If there isn't, you need to allow them to get Jessica to surgery without delay. Time is critical."

I pull my eyes from the elevator to focus on the woman. I expect her to look stern and forceful, but her features are soft, and her kind eyes search my face.

"I understand," I assure her. "Thank you."

"Once we are on the surgical floor, I can show you to the waiting area."

"Can I follow her to surgery? I want to stay with her as long as I can."

"We'll see once we get upstairs." She moves away from the double doors just in time. A gurney bursts through them, surrounded by doctors and nurses. Jessica lies still in the middle of them all, and my heart is in my throat, but I call to her as quickly as I can.

"I'm here, baby. Mommy's here. You are going to be fine."

She's gone as quickly as she came. While we wait for the CT scan to be performed, I review the plan with the woman. Such a simple plan, with easy instructions, but I'm still afraid of being lost in a hospital maze, unable to find my daughter again.

After what feels like an eternity, my girl is in the hallway, still surrounded by doctors and nurses, and I'm running to keep up with them, determined to make it into the elevator. As we pile in, I move to the head of the gurney and lean in close to Jessica.

"You are going to be fine." I repeat the mantra I began in the dirt at the barn. "The doctors are going to take really good care of you, and you are going to be fine."

Too soon, the elevator doors open, and they whisk Jessica away. I follow until the dreaded words are delivered: "This is as far as you can go."

I stay rooted to the spot outside the surgical ward, trying to watch through the crack between the doors as they rush my girl away from me again.

The short woman and Jim Williams appear. "Ms. Lavine, we can show you to the waiting area." I nod and follow them, looking for Becky.

"Where is . . . ?"

"We've told your friend where you'll be."

"My husband is on his way. How do I tell him where I am?"

"Anyone coming to be with you should go to the emergency room lobby, and we will direct them to you here."

We reach a small waiting room that I hope is reserved for our family alone. There are a couple of tables holding magazines and informational pamphlets and a dozen chairs, but that's it. Windows look out onto a courtyard. I'm surprised to see the sun is still shining.

I pull out my phone to text Jesse before collapsing into one of the chairs. The woman sits beside me and finally introduces herself. "My name is Grace, and I am a social worker here at the hospital. Jim and I are here to support you in any way we can."

"Thank you. How long will it be before they come to give us an update?"

"That all depends on how your daughter's surgery goes. Can you tell me what happened?"

I shake my head as I see Becky returning with her husband, Steve. "I'm unsure of the details myself. All I know is she was kicked in the head by a horse. I don't know how it happened." Becky and Steve hug me before sitting down on the opposite side of the small room.

Grace points out the phone on the wall and tells me the extension to dial if we need anything. She excuses herself to check on other patients.

Moments later, I spot Kari coming down the hall. She hugs me tight then sits next to me, grabs my hand and squeezes hard. "It's going to be okay."

Is it?

I try to slow my mind.

Of course it is. One way or another, it has to be.

I squeeze Kari's hand in response and fumble through introductions.

I check my phone. There are no messages from Jesse, so I send another message to him: *Are you close?*

"Is Jesse on his way?" Kari asks.

I hold up my phone. "I'm trying to find out where he is. He had to go to the barn to get Jocelyn first. He should be here any minute, though." I check the time on the phone and try to calculate the amount of time Jesse will need to travel from his office to the barn and then to the hospital. Simple math involving roads I have traveled hundreds of times, yet I can't wrap my head around the navigation.

"I don't know. I don't know where he is."

"He'll be here." She pats my leg. As if on cue, he walks into the waiting area, carrying a still-sleeping Jocelyn. I jump up to hug him as best I can without waking Jocelyn. I am envious of her ability to sleep through the chaos.

Kari switches seats so Jesse can sit next to me. Soon the energy surrounding us settles enough for my breathing to return to normal.

Grace and Jim return to assess the situation. Jim sits next to Jesse as Grace introduces herself to everyone.

"Do you follow a particular religion?" the chaplain finally asks. Jesse and I exchange a quick glance before he answers for both of us.

"Not any particular one, no. We don't belong to a church, but we practice our own beliefs." I'm relieved that Jim doesn't push him for more. Instead, he reiterates his role of companion and supporter for the family. Something we will gladly accept.

"So..." Grace starts gingerly, looking at me and glancing around the room, "can you tell me what happened now?"

"I...I don't know." I look at Becky. If this were any other situation, and I were watching as an outsider, I wouldn't even think to press her for details. The shock is apparent on her face; she is clinging to Steve as tightly as I am holding onto Kari and Jesse. If the situation were any different, I would let her collect herself and worry about details another day.

But this isn't any other situation. I am not an outsider. My daughter is in surgery, and I have no clue why.

"What happened?" I ask as gently as I can, hoping she understands that I'm not accusing her of anything.

"I don't know myself. We had barely gotten to the pasture to put the lead on Katie and take her to the barn when Tinkerbell came running down from the treat pasture. There was no reason for her to be there. She had already been ridden and groomed and was up in the pasture with the good grass. She should have been eating, but she came running into the area, wanting to be ridden again. She went to kick Katie out of the way, but Katie moved. That left Jessica unprotected. It all happened so fast."

"I know it did," I say softly. "We couldn't have been there very long before it happened. It had to have been seconds. I am sure she will be fine. Hopefully, they'll be able to tell us something soon. In the meantime, I'd better go call Melissa."

Searching my phone for Melissa's number, I head into the hallway. Melissa has been Jessica's dance instructor for the past seven years. She is the head coach of the competition team Jessica dances with, and they are supposed to have a dress rehearsal tonight for their last competition of the season.

No, not only the last competition of the season but the last competition for this particular dance company. Melissa is leaving for another studio next year. Jessica will be so disappointed to have missed the final competition. With shaky hands, I dial Melissa's number.

"Hello?"

"Melissa?"

"Yes?"

"It's Jolene, Jessica's mom."

"Hi! How are you?"

"I've been better. There was an accident at Jessica's barn today. Jessica won't be at rehearsal tonight or at competition this weekend."

"Excuse me?"

I am thrown off by the shock in her voice and try to reassure her.

"I am sure she will be fine," I repeat for the hundredth time today. "She is in surgery now, and we haven't received an update or seen a doctor yet."

"What is she in surgery for? Is she okay?"

"I'm sure she is. She was kicked in the head, but we got to the hospital very quickly, so I'm sure she will be fine."

"Okay..." she doesn't sound sure, and I search for the right words to reassure her.

"I'll call you as soon as I hear anything, but can you tell everyone why we're gone? I'll send an email to the dance list as soon as I find out what's going on."

"Okay, I will. Give her our love."

"I definitely will."

I hang up the phone and look down the corridor, searching for a doctor who might be able to give us an update. The hallway is deserted, so I return to our little corner of the hospital.

"How'd that go?" Jesse asks.

I shrug. "I think maybe I should have waited. I didn't have much information to give, except that we wouldn't be there and why. She sounded really worried."

"Yeah, I wish they would come and tell us something. How long has it been?"

I check the time on my phone and find I'm having trouble with basic math functions again. "I don't know. I'm not sure what time we got here or how long I was waiting before surgery. I don't have a real great sense of time right now."

"Well, you called me at 2:00. My conference call had just started."

"And we got to the barn at 1:45. I called you as we were getting in the ambulance. Wow." I shake my head and look at Becky. "It really was seconds, wasn't it?"

She can only nod, and I continue the timeline.

"We got to the barn at 1:45 and finished our conversation..." The force of the last conversation I had with Jessica hits me, and I'm crying for the first time since we pulled into the barn.

"Oh, honey." Jesse tries to pull me to him, but Jocelyn's sleeping body blocks him.

Kari jumps up. "Let me have her. I'll walk around for a little bit, and when she wakes up, I'll go to the cafeteria. Do you want anything?"

I shake my head, "Maybe just something to drink."

"Okay, I'll be back in a bit." As she walks through the door, Jesse, now unencumbered, holds me tight.

"It's going to be okay," he says to reassure me.

"I hope you're right," I whisper as I try to breathe and stay grounded.

CHAPTER FOUR

I Broke All the Rules

May 1999

I never wanted children.

I know I'm not the first person to deal with seemingly insurmountable obstacles as a child. I have definitely heard more horrific and sordid tales than my own. But the bottom line is that the difficult parts of my childhood didn't leave a gentle mark on my soul.

I entered my adult years without the coping skills, common sense, or art of perspective needed to handle day-to-day life, let alone any major life change. I was petrified of being a bad mother. Unwilling to put my issues onto a child and clueless about how I could prevent transferring my baggage to an unsuspecting soul, I felt unqualified to raise another human being.

From the time I was sixteen, I'd been on the pill and had never given it a second thought. In my mid twenties, I realized there had to be a reason for how sick I was feeling and how irregular my periods had become.

I embraced denial long enough to hold the birthday celebration I'd planned for my good friend Jesse but couldn't avoid the fact that the incense and cigarette smoke from the party turned my stomach.

In the week following the party, I tried to detox. I gave up my numerous vices and slept. A lot. When those tactics failed to heal me, I called my best friend, Kari, to ask for advice. A dozen years into our friendship at that point, I didn't need to say much before she understood my predicament and headed to my house, stopping at the drugstore on the way.

When she arrived, there was little conversation before I disappeared into the bathroom. I didn't have enough time to set a timer or even pull up my pants before the obvious answer to my question glared at me from the white stick sitting on the bathroom sink.

I returned to the living room and held out the test for Kari to see. She instantly threw her arms around me and shouted gleefully, "You're going to have a baby!"

I hugged her back, clutching at her for support as my mind raced to remember all the abuse I'd put my body through. Pot, alcohol, cigarettes, late nights, early mornings, screaming fights, too much sleep, not enough sleep…not to mention the fact that I was on the pill.

How can I be pregnant?

I sat on the couch and tried to breathe. Kari sat next to me, grabbed my hand, and squeezed hard. "It's going to be okay."

Was it?

I tried to slow my mind.

Of course it is. One way or another, it has to be.

Kari squeezed my hand again. "Honey?"

I sighed and met her eyes, touched by the concern reflected back at me.

"Are you okay?"

I nodded and hugged her again, trying to comprehend how much my life was about to change.

CHAPTER FIVE

Glimpses of Truth Thou Hast for Me

"Mr. and Mrs. Lavine?"

I feel like Angels are singing and the light has descended from on high. The doctor has finally entered the room.

"Yes," we reply in unison as we jump up to greet him.

"I'm Dr. Bosco. Your daughter is still in surgery, but I wanted to give you an update that we have gotten her stabilized."

"So, she'll be okay?"

"I can't tell you that right now. Her injury was very severe. We have gotten her stable, and they are still working on her. It may be another hour or two."

"Wait. I'm confused. If she is stable, she is going to be okay, right?"

The doctor holds his hands up as if to block my eagerness for a positive response. He scowls at me, repeating his earlier words. "I'm not able to tell you that right now. I'll come back when her surgery is done."

I watch him exit the room, mouth agape.

"What the hell?" Jesse voices my confusion.

"I'm glad I'm not the only one with that reaction. *What the hell* is right. If she is stable, then she will be okay. Right?"

Grace has returned, her arms filled with coloring books, crayons, and toys for Jocelyn. She takes one look at us and drops everything onto a seat.

"I saw Dr. Bosco in the hall. Did he speak with you?"

"If you can call it that." I drop back into the chair, looking out the window.

"He's a brilliant doctor," she says to reassure us. "He just isn't warm and fuzzy."

"That's an understatement. He seemed annoyed that I had the nerve to ask for some good news regarding my child's health. That's all I wanted."

"Until the surgery is done, he won't be able to tell you much."

I continue to stare out the window, trying to shake the uneasy feeling that is growing inside me.

"She is going to be fine." The words escape in an exhale, barely louder than a whisper.

"What, honey?" Jesse sits down and pulls me close to him.

"She is going to be fine." It's not much louder than the first time I said it, and he simply raises his eyebrows and glances at the social worker.

I turn to him and take his face in my hands.

"She is going to be fine," I whisper again. "The Angels said it, so it must be true."

Jesse closes his eyes and touches his forehead to mine.

"She is going to be fine," he whispers.

She is going to be fine.

"I don't know why I let you talk me into this," I barked at Jesse as I struggled to navigate the dark forest road.

"You told me some of your best memories as a kid were of camping. I didn't realize you needed to be talked into this trip."

"I guess I should have been more specific then."

I couldn't decide if I felt more angry or scared, so I shook my head and gripped the steering wheel tighter, trying to concentrate on the ground in front of the car.

Jesse had a point. My family's annual summer camping trips to various forests in Northern California were some of the few events of my childhood I remember with pure joy. The time spent hiking through the big trees, rafting down the river rapids, and sleeping under the stars instilled in me a love of the outdoors. Communing with nature helped me the find peace and comfort that was missing from so much of my day-to-day life growing up.

Being able to share that experience with my best friend, with whom I was not-so-secretly hoping to move to the next level, should have been an opportunity I jumped at.

The conflict I felt when he broached the subject of a new weekend activity resulted from knowledge I had *because* I spent so much time in those woods growing up. I knew better than to go camping on one of the most notoriously busy recreational weekends of the year: Labor Day.

Jesse pleaded his case, insisting that we would be able to find something, even if it wasn't the best spot. After all, the Crystal Basin Recreational Area in the El Dorado National Forest boasts more than seven hundred developed campsites. He might have been right if we hadn't left at 7:00 on Friday night. However, since I was eager to have alone time with Jesse away from the large group of friends we usually partied with, I succumbed to his weak argument.

That'll teach me.

Of course all of the developed campgrounds were booked, so we ended up looking for a more rustic campground Jesse remembered visiting as a young child. That meant we had to drive on a road that was less road and more rocks and dirt. Although surrounded by the gigantic trees I so love, I couldn't even enjoy the view, thanks to the rain and the moonless night.

To make matters worse, my beloved Honda Prelude was not the best vehicle for the adventure. Front-end damage had left it with only one headlight that functioned (and barely, at that), and the windshield wipers were creating streaks.

Two of my fears were driving at night and getting lost. Add rain to the mix, and I was torn between making my way through the darkness in order to spend more time with Jesse and heading home to curl up in front of a roaring fire, which is how I prefer to take my stormy nights.

I struggled to keep my fear in check and resist the urge to snap at Jesse again. Instead, I leaned forward, struggling to see through the windshield into the dark night beyond.

"Well," Jesse said gently, "we obviously took a wrong turn."

I inhaled deeply and tried to glare at him out of the corner of my eye. "Are you sure? You said the site was in the middle of nowhere. We're certainly in the middle of nowhere now."

"Yes, we are." Jesse carefully measured his words and made a point to crane his neck to look out the window at the darkened sky. "I just... it's dark, it's late—"

"You think? If only *someone* had warned us about trying to go camping at such a late hour on such a busy weekend. If only *someone* had the benefit of years of camping experience to draw upon. If only—"

He finally snapped back at me. "Okay! You were right. I thought it would be a good place to have some time alone, away from our friends, to finally figure out what the hell we're doing."

My anger and fear were swiftly replaced by the embarrassing realization that my "oblivious" best friend had finally picked up the hints I'd dropped about wanting to be more than friends. My temper tantrum was in danger of ruining all of my hoped-for progress.

"Oh." I was simply amazed at my brilliant response.

"Yeah. Obviously, I'm just a city kid who has no idea of the ways of this world, so I'll keep my mouth shut now, and you, Ms. Wilderness Mountain Woman, can work to get us out of here."

I bit my lip and struggled to concentrate on the road. I didn't think it was possible for me to drive any slower, but I took my foot completely off the gas, glanced at Jesse again, and silently began calling on my Angels.

About a year before, I'd been shopping at a metaphysical store in Folsom, California, called Planet Earth Rising and had purchased a small box of Angel cards. The cards were small, only about two inches wide and three-quarters of an inch tall. Instead of the typical Angel names, such as Michael, Gabriel, or Raphael, those cards depicted attributes. Words like Truth, Play, and Adventure were printed on the fifty-two cards, each naming a nondescript Angel (or Angels) acting out their assigned attribute.

I'd been working with the cards since then, meditating with them and creating my own bit of sacred space. I'd talk with them about everything from the *Big Traumatic Stuff* I felt a constant struggle to move past to the petty drama of day-to-day life. The small stuff might not have been as worthy of Angelic meditations, but petty arguments and supposed offenses were definitely easier to focus on.

That night, sitting in the middle of a forest in the pouring rain, arguing with my best friend and feeling scared out of my mind, seemed to be the moment all of those meditations were leading up to.

Angels, Angels all around. Angels, Angels, come surround. Guys? I could really use some help here. Can I get a sign if I'm driving in the wrong direction? Maybe a rock or a tree branch or something?

"Hey, are you okay?" Jesse's voice startled me back to reality, and I realized that I'd dropped further into meditation than I'd intended and we'd stalled out.

"Yeah, sorry, I was..." I restarted the car and chose my words carefully. "I was asking for help."

His features softened, and I inched the car forward again.

"Your Angels?"

"Yeah. I asked them for some sort of sign we're going the wrong way. Something like a rock or a tree branch to point us in the right direction."

He studied the road ahead of us. "Like that rock?"

"No, I need something more obvious."

We crept along as I struggled to put away my pride and determination and simply turn around.

"Tree branch!" Jesse pointed out the limb hanging over the road.

"Which way is it pointing? Do we keep going or go back?"

Jesse fixed me with a gaze that was equal parts perplexed, exasperated, and impatient. "Okay, let me in on the secret here. Exactly how much will you question the directionality of the tree branches before you turn around?"

"I don't know. I'll know it when I see it." I spoke carefully, trying to remember that he and I hadn't had a complete meeting of the minds regarding my spiritual beliefs. He'd been open to the pieces I've shared bit by bit, but that night's adventure seemed to push the envelope.

"I realize I'm new to this, but it seems to me if you've asked for help to know when it's time to turn around, then a big rock or a tree branch or . . . I don't know . . . *the car stalling out* should be a big, shining sign. How much longer do you want to be out here?"

"I know." I sighed, unable to argue with his logic. "We've already been out here for hours as it is."

"Well, I wouldn't say hours."

To prove my point, I reached out and moved the maps and packing lists that had blocked the dashboard clock.

"Forty-five minutes." He made the statement with a touch too much smugness in his voice.

"Oh, shut it."

I returned my attention to the road just in time to scream and slam on the brakes. Jesse yelled too, slamming on the imaginary brake on his side of the car and grabbing for the dashboard.

We had to run out of road-that's-not-a-road eventually, but the sudden appearance of an enormous boulder, too big to drive around, was shocking nonetheless. Had I been driving any faster than a crawl, we surely would have crashed.

After the few heart-racing moments it took us to catch our breath, Jesse reached over, very gently took my hand and whispered, "Should we get out and climb over, or is it time to head back to civilization?"

I forced a laugh and began the laborious task of turning around.

Under normal circumstances, a three-point turnabout would have gotten us out of the mess. That night, the three-point turnabout easily morphed into a thirty-three-point turnabout in the darkness. I mumbled pleas and gratitude to the Angels the whole time.

Once I finally navigated the complete 180 degrees, I sat for a minute, willing my heart rate to return to normal. Even though the moon had momentarily emerged from the clouds, I dreaded having to head back down the muddy road we had already traveled.

"Should we go?" Jesse asked breathlessly.

"Yeah, I just..." As though in a trance, I took a moment to open my door and look out.

"What are you doing?" Jesse grabbed my arm and reached over me to grab the door. In the same moment, I slammed it shut, muttering a collection of expletives under my breath.

"Why did you do that? What were you hoping to see?"

"Not *that*." My voice too shrill for the small confines of the car.

"What did you see?" he asked as he loosened his grip on my arm.

"Nothing." I exhaled and closed my eyes.

"No, seriously, what?"

"No, seriously." I opened my eyes and looked at him directly. "Nothing. No road. No shoulder. Just a drop-off down the side of the mountain."

Before I could even think about how we should already have fallen off the side of the mountain, I was pulled into a trance again, and a vision of little Angels hung above my head.

Sitting in my broken-down car on the side of a mountain on a dark and stormy night, I began to realize exactly how real the Angels had become to me. My heart was in my throat. Although I tried to take a deep, calming breath, it was no use. The tears were falling.

"Hey, what's wrong? We're okay. We just gotta drive the other way now. We're going to be okay."

"I know," I wailed, "but we shouldn't be! We should have plummeted to a fiery death by now."

He chuckled at me, and I shook my head.

"I'm sure in the past you've thought I was crazy with the Angel stuff..."

"I don't think you're crazy, it's just... it's your thing."

"Well, I may step fully into crazy now. I've been talking to my Angels since I asked for help."

"Okay, and...?"

"They sent me a vision."

He raised his eyebrows and cocked his head.

"I have no idea why I opened the door to look out. I felt compelled to do it, and I'm not kidding: there is nothing there. No road or shoulder. Only the drop-off. As soon as I closed the door, I received a vision of the car floating halfway off the mountain, hanging over the precipice, with those cute little Angels from my cards holding the car up as I turned the wheel."

Jesse slumped into his seat and stared out the windshield. "But there has to be something."

"Do you want to look?"

I pushed my seat back to give him enough space to lean over me. After grabbing hold of the emergency brake between the seats, I opened the door so he could look out. He hesitated for a minute before taking off his seatbelt and crawling over to confirm my story. I lightly touched his leg and breathed in the scent of his cologne before he slid back to his seat.

"Well?" I studied his features.

He cleared his throat and turned to face me. "So, how many Angels were holding up the car?"

I exhaled with a small laugh before crying again. He grabbed me into a tight hug and whispered in my ear, "Let's get out of here."

I squeezed him back, taking a moment to enjoy the intimacy, before steeling myself for another forty-five minute drive.

As we made our way out of the wilderness, I offered up prayers of gratitude to the Angelic beings I'd imagined dancing on miniature cards. That night they became bigger than life to keep us safe in a way I never knew or imagined was possible.

I truly believe we owe them our lives.

Grace pulls Jesse and me from our shared memory to tell us the doctor will see us now.

Before we leave the waiting room, I lose myself in Jesse's arms again. "I heard their voices when I was lying in the dirt with Jessica," I whisper to him. "They were surrounding us with their wings. It's their words I am repeating."

"She will be fine?"

"Yes. I've been talking to them since arriving at the hospital, begging them to work more of their magic. I hope they can keep us from driving off the cliff again."

We reach a conference room at the end of the hall and see Jim already seated. Grace takes the seat next to him, and we sit on the opposite side of the table. Dr. Bosco enters a few minutes later and positions himself at the end of the conference table.

I'm struck by his relaxed posture as he leans back in his chair, crossing one leg over the other. He begins to speak, but I don't follow anything he is saying except for the parts I'm trying to hear. The surgery went well, Jessica is stable, and they are waiting for the anesthesia to wear off. Everything else he says may as well be Greek. I can't take my eyes off my fingers, which are intertwined with Jesse's on the table.

Jesse asks a couple of questions, and I try to ignore the doctor's exasperation this time. He is picking at the edge of the table and seems to be using the same words to answer every question Jesse asks. Finally, he repeats the same thing he told us in the waiting room. "That's all I can tell you for now. That's all I have."

He stands up and leaves the room without another word. I feel stunned.

"Will he be back?"

Jim and Grace exchange a knowing look, and I press them for more information. "Is he usually like this?"

Jim bows his head, and Grace offers a weak response. "He's an excellent doctor..."

"He very well may be, but I don't understand anything he said." I plead with her. "What is happening?"

Jesse pulls me toward him and holds me close. He has obviously listened better than I did, as he asks more specific questions. "He mentioned they might be transferring us. Is that happening?"

"That part we can tell you. Yes. They plan to transfer Jessica to the children's hospital."

"UCD?" I ask, not trusting the feeling of relief that seems to be creeping in. *How can I be relieved when we don't have any answers?*

"Yes. UC Davis Children's Hospital. You know where it is?"

"Of course I know where it is. It's the best hospital in the region." Once I've spoken the words, my sense of relief makes more sense. UC Davis Medical Center is a world-renowned teaching hospital with a stellar Pediatric Intensive Care Unit. I am relieved that we are being sent to the best children's hospital in the region, while simultaneously feeling shock that one of my children is sick enough to need the best children's hospital in the region.

Darkness threatens to overwhelm me as Jesse and I follow Jim and Grace to the ICU, where Jessica is recovering from surgery. We wait at the doors to the intensive care wing for what feels like an eternity, and then we're there, at her bedside. Three nurses move in and out and about her room, opening packages and hooking up monitors.

"You can talk to her," Chris, the nurse, tells me. "She's coming out of the anesthesia now. We'll determine the next steps after it wears off."

"What do you mean?" The question is automatic, as I'm mesmerized by the sight of Jessica in the hospital bed. She seems to instinctively turn toward her left side, as if she is aware of the wound that covers the right side of her head.

"Her turning like that means she is responding to stimuli."

I almost ask what he means again, but I see that he is holding a metal instrument in one hand, and his other hand is still on Jessica's foot.

"She was able to feel that." To further make his point, he comes to the head of her bed and pinches her shoulders, causing Jessica to instinctively pull away again.

"Okay. I understand," I tell him quickly, wanting him to leave her alone.

"We will be watching her vitals for . . ." His voice trails off, as I'm floating with the Angels again.

She will be fine.

CHAPTER SIX

And I Am Beside You

I don't understand what's going on. I've woken up from the shortest and most disjointed sleep I've ever had. While I feel awake in the sense that I can't imagine being able to fall back asleep, my head feels foggy and things are moving in slow motion.

Feeling around the chair that served as my bed last night, I search for my phone. Sleeping in the chair isn't as uncomfortable as it sounds. It's a larger chair with two sections that pull out, so it becomes what some might call a bed. Okay, it's exactly as uncomfortable as it sounds.

I eventually find my phone on the floor under the chair, and my mind clears enough to remember talking to Kari until the early morning hours. I must have fallen asleep mid-conversation, as I don't remember saying goodbye to her. I check to see if Jesse has texted or called yet, but no messages greet me. It's 6:30 a.m. I probably got about three hours of sleep last night.

The transfer from Sutter to UCD involved discussions about whether to take a helicopter or an ambulance and then parades of nurses and paramedics through the maze of back exits and entrances for two hospitals. I remember looking at the stars briefly before I climbed into the front seat of the ambulance, but I don't remember if Kari, Jesse, and Jocelyn followed us here, or if it's been just Jessica and me since arriving at UCD.

I sit and watch the people move around the nurse's station outside Jessica's room. It's been a long time since I've been in a hospital, but it seems to me there are more people milling about than usual.

Eventually, Marcy, Jessica's nurse, enters, followed by a man with short brown hair and a goatee. Marcy motions toward my girl, who is "sleeping" in the bed, and begins to introduce us to her coworker. "This is Jessica and her mom..."

"Jolene," I remind her, standing up and offering my hand.

"Right, Jolene. This is Erik, and he'll be taking over for me."

"It's nice to meet you, Erik. Thank you."

"It's nice to meet you, too. I'll be back to do my assessments and talk to you in a bit."

Nodding, I set my phone down and make my way to the bed, where Jessica is covered in too many wires to count. I touch her head gently and whisper to her the song that I've sung to wake her up since she was a toddler. "Good morning, good morning, it's a great day to be alive. Good morning, good morning to you, you, a boo ba di do. I'm so glad you're alive. I love you."

How did we get here? We should be at home, sleeping in, getting plenty of rest to prepare for her last dance competition of the year. I simply stare at her.

My thoughts are interrupted by people moving in and out of her room. Doctors, nurses, and... more doctors? Some are in the typical white coats, some of them are in scrubs, and some are wearing both. I don't know who is who or why so many are coming and going, checking the computer that monitors Jessica's vital signs and the IVs that hang to the left of her bed.

Overwhelmed by the number of IVs, I wonder how many she is actually hooked up to. There are two different types of machines hanging on the IV poles, but they all have tubes coming from them, with lights flashing and different sets of numbers on the displays.

Breaking the machines down into rows and columns makes it easier to ignore the tubes and beeping. I fall back on a counting trick I use to calm myself and determine a concrete answer that doesn't help calm my nerves much.

Seventeen.

She couldn't possibly be hooked up to that many IVs.

I look down at her and try to take it all in. Wires and tubes come out of her from head to toe. Where could seventeen IVs lead? Some tubes look like they have more than one port, and others are secured by bandages and medical tape. I can't tell where one IV ends and the next begins. I think I can see connections in each foot and possibly another in her ankle, as well as one in her right arm and maybe her left wrist. I can't tell if there is actually an IV on the back of her hand, or if it's only a bandage.

Feeling a little dizzy, I realize I'm holding my breath and force myself to slowly exhale. My head is still foggy, and I am desperate for answers. I don't know which of the doctors or nurses to talk to as they cluster outside the glass door, talking in hushed tones.

I try to remember to breathe as I look around at the rest of the room. There is a sink behind the IV poles, a fluorescent light bar above the head of the bed, and another machine, which I think is a ventilator, on the right. The wall to the right of the bed is mostly windows, across which the curtains are drawn, blocking out the rising sun. My chair-bed hybrid sits under the windows, along with a standard chair for visitors. The other walls hold bulletin boards and medical notices. To the left of my chair-bed are receptacles for linens, trash, and biohazard, as well as a cabinet that is probably supposed to serve as a nightstand. That is where my purse sits, along with the hospital phone and my cell.

In the center of it all, of course, is the bed. I study Jessica again, trying to see more than IV tubes. A cervical collar has been placed around her neck. A tube goes into her nose, and her left arm is splinted. She's wearing some sort of cuffs on her legs, and her face is covered with surgical tape that holds the ventilator in place.

Then there's her head. It is difficult for me to look at her head. I reach out to lightly touch it, but there are so many bandages and a tube coming out the right side of her skull. I am afraid of bumping her and injuring her or moving any of the wires that might make the machines start screaming at me.

Her long, beautiful brown hair is a mess of curls and tangles on the pillow.

The only part of the scene that seems even remotely normal is her Thomy bear, a Teddy bear she received for her fourth birthday. It's her favorite and most trusted ally. Amidst the chaos of phone calls and waiting rooms that followed the accident, I had enough clarity to ask for some comfort items from home for her.

Thomy has fallen halfway through the bedrail and is dangling close to the floor. I pull him up and gently place him next to Jessica's chest. Tied around Thomy is the yellow baby blanket Jessica has had since she was three years old, inside of which is tucked a small memento of my dad. I place my hand on these treasures, thinking about the love Jessica has poured into them. If the whimsical fairy tales of a child's love bringing favorite toys to life might possibly be true, I imagine Thomy gathering that love and strength and returning it to Jessica.

Erik has returned and begins typing into the computer.

"How is she?" I ask softly.

"The doctors are doing their rounds right now. I've asked them to come and look at her numbers." His voice is clipped, quick, and professional, and his eyes never leave the computer screen.

"I saw. They've been in and out."

"I hope they'll be able to tell you something soon. I'm sorry; I'll be right back." He takes some notes and pushes through the door. He talks quickly to the doctors clustered outside.

I check my phone again, with the same result. No messages. I hate to wake Jesse and Jocelyn, not knowing how late they were here last night, but the longer I'm awake and standing in this room alone, seeing the doctors move in and out, the more I feel panic rising up in me.

I don't know what is going on.

I need my husband.

I pick up the phone and dial his cell. It rolls to voicemail, so I call the home number, which Jesse answers on the third ring. I finally grasp the full meaning of the saying "my port in the storm." I find it a little easier to breathe now that we've connected.

"I'm sorry to wake you. Is Jocelyn still asleep? When are you coming back?"

"I just got out of the shower and am getting ready to get Jocelyn up and take her to daycare. Then I'll be on my way."

"Okay." I can't take my eyes off the doctors as I try to keep my voice calm. "Something seems to be happening. A new nurse is here, and there seem to be an excessive number of doctors. I need you."

"How is Jess?"

"I don't know. She seems the same to me, but I don't know what I'm looking for, and–"

At that moment, I'm interrupted by a group of doctors stepping in. "Ms. Lavine?"

"Yes."

"I'm Dr. Harlan, I'm a resident here. This is Dr. Kerr, a neurosurgery resident, and Joan is our neurosurgery nurse practitioner. Is your husband here, as well?"

"No. I'm talking to him now." I speak slowly, and my eyes follow Dr. Kerr and Joan as they shine a light in Jessica's eyes, check the computer, and speak softly to one another. They look at the dressing that covers the damage to the right side of her head.

"Is he on his way here?"

"We were just discussing it . . . is . . . how is . . . ? Is Jessica okay?"

"It would be wise for your husband to be here."

"What does that mean?" I put the phone up to my mouth again. "Honey, the doctors are here. They say you need to be here."

"No, Ms. Lavine." The doctor gets my attention again. "*Anyone* who needs to be here, needs to be here now."

This doctor can't possibly know what he is talking about. Jessica is going to be fine.

"Did you hear that?" I asked Jesse.

"No, what did he say?"

I try to telepathically convey the message, not wanting to give spoken power to the doctor's words. I look over at the doctors examining Jessica and back to Dr. Harlan.

"Ms. Lavine?"

"He said anyone who needs to be here, needs to be here now. They still haven't told me what's happening, but call everyone and get here as soon as you can."

I hear the sharp intake of his breath then, "Okay. I love you."

"I love you, too." I hang up and close my eyes for a second.

When I open them, Nurse Practitioner Joan turns to me and begins saying lots of big words that sound very serious. Her voice crashes over me, and I stare at her dumbly, desperate to understand what she is telling me.

The doctors eventually leave the room, and I sit on the edge of the chair and stare at my daughter. It doesn't take long for me to realize my Angels have returned, and I begin to rub my hands together.

CHAPTER SEVEN

There Now, Steady Love

I didn't believe in much in my youth. The majority of my experiences with church and those who believe in God and Jesus were so full of hypocrisy, judgment, and emotional trauma that for many years I didn't bother with the trappings of church and organized religion.

Some people who knew me then are quick to tell you tales of my disrespect: the rolling of eyes whenever God or prayer were mentioned or how I would bristle if someone said "God Bless You" when I sneezed. The funny thing is those who so readily offer evidence of the ignorance of my youth are just as quick to mock my beliefs as an adult, usually referring to them as "whatever you believe in this week."

Like many others, my beliefs are complex. I don't believe in a set of rules handed down from a mountain. I don't believe in the God of my youth, a guy sitting on an ornate throne in a cloudy, ethereal Heaven, scepter in one hand and checklist in the other.

I don't believe He is watching over me to determine if I pray too little, cuss too much, or enjoy sex a little too often. I don't believe I will be sent to hell for petty thoughts about inane subjects.

It's difficult for me to believe in a God with a set of rules so long and detailed that men on Earth still can't agree on them or stop killing one another in His name.

Despite all of that, I can find beauty in parts of many different religions. I believe in Angelic beings. I believe in treating people with respect and kindness, because it is the right thing to do and not because I'm afraid of burning for all eternity.

I believe in . . . well . . . physics, basically. I believe that all things are made up of energy, including people and their thoughts. To that end, I believe our thoughts become our reality, but phrasing it as such oversimplifies the process.

I don't believe in coincidence; I do believe in signs. I believe in reincarnation and Karma, and I've been practicing *The Secret* since 1996. *The Secret* is really not much of one. It's high school physics: For every action, there is *always* an equal and opposite reaction. Put good out; get good back.

I believe in the Light and the Dark and the Beauty that can be found in the Balance of The Universe. I believe when born of Love, all paths lead to the same Source.

I usually find *my* path when sitting in the forest, surrounded by giant trees that are thousands of years old, or when relaxing on the beach, unable to see where the ocean ends and the sky begins. In those moments, I feel I'm one with The Universe, but only if I remember the Beauty of The Universe is inside me. It's inside all of us.

Even though I realize how insignificant we all are in the light of eternity, we're often told that our presence, our actions, and even our mere thoughts can make a difference. Perhaps it is the depth of the human connection that I believe in most of all.

To put it simply, "what I believe in this week" is most accurately summed up in the portion of a Venn diagram where science and magic intersect. When I'm fortunate enough to locate the balance between those two points, I feel that I've found where the mystery ends and the magic begins.

I'm teetering between those two places right now.

In this cold hospital room, monitors beep and voices sound rushed and desperate, but I'm oblivious to most of them as I simply rub my hands together.

From the moment I slid into the dirt next to Jessica, whispering, "You will be fine," I have not let my thoughts waver from that outcome. But now I can't even understand my own thoughts, let alone what's going on at the nurse's station just outside the door of Jessica's room. Something has changed, and I don't know what it is.

All I can think to do is pray. Manifest. Meditate. Chant. Through whatever terms are acceptable and to whatever forces will listen. Mystery or magic, God or Angels, or just the cumulative years of cold, hard science these doctors have studied so hard to master. Whatever the secret is, I'm calling on it now.

Because I'm not a doctor or a nurse, I don't know how to make sense of the numbers on the screen that seem to be the source of everyone's frenzied state. Instead, I hope to connect with what I do know. My Baby Girl. My little Mini-Me. My sweet Sunshine Girl, who is lying in a bed, covered in wires and tubes. On that bed, in the midst of all those wires, something is going wrong.

I rub my hands together a little faster and begin to chant. "Angels, Angels all around, Angels, Angels, please surround..."

She will be fine. She has to be. No matter how deep the coma, she will be fine. No matter how grave the looks on the doctors' faces, she will be fine. Jesse is on his way. He will be able to figure everything out, and she will be fine.

I'm rubbing my hands together faster now. As the heat from the friction grows, a fog overwhelms me, shutting out the increasing chaos and commotion.

I imagine a thread of white light coming down from the ether, entering my body at the crown of my head. I imagine a second thread of light, green this time, coming up from Mother Earth and entering my body through the soles of my feet.

I feel myself floating to Jessica's bedside, where I hold my hands over her damaged head. "You are healing," I whisper to her, slowly at first, and then faster and faster, until my voice finds a chanting rhythm. "You are healing, you are healing, you are healing, you are healing."

The mystery ends.

The magic begins.

Positioned beside my daughter's hospital bed with my eyes closed and a rush of blood drowning out the doctors' and nurses' urgency, I see the Light and Love I have asked for flowing toward Jessica's body.

In the early hours of that morning, sleep had evaded me. I was at a loss as to what to do next, so I sent an email to Jessica's Dance Company, her Girl Scout troop, and numerous friends and loved ones, telling them what happened and asking them to do whatever they could to raise her name in healing. I didn't care whether that meant praying or sending energy, thinking good thoughts, lighting candles, or dancing around the campfire shaking tambourines. I asked for whatever thoughts and energy they could spare.

They have answered my call in full force.

I am vaguely aware of Jesse's arrival and the doctors and nurses entering the room again. Insistent voices raised in disagreement threaten to pull me from my trance. It sounds as if everyone is speaking a foreign language, and the only thing I understand is the urgency and the tension. These people are not on the same page.

I desperately switch things up, pleading with all that is holy, everything from Allah to Zeus, The Universe, Spirit, God, Buddha, Ra, Source, Creator, The One. To whomever will listen, I plead, "Let the doctors' path be lit; let the choices be clear. Remove all obstacles; let the path be clear. One clear voice; let this be heard. One *true* voice; let this be heard. In Light and Love and in harmony with The Universe. You are healing. Let this be heard."

I feel as though I am dissolving into The Universe, and I breathe with the waves of energy soaring toward Jessica now. I envision the Light, Love, and prayers of those we have called upon to send up healing for our sweet girl, and I harness all of this energy and direct it into her precious head. All the while I continue to chant: "You are healing; let the path be lit; you are healing; let the choices be clear; you are healing; let this be heard. You are healing."

Discord and aggressive energy once again threaten to pull me back to reality, and I realize I'm no longer next to Jessica. Panic begins to rise up when I open my eyes enough to see that I'm now on the bench in the hall outside her room. Family and friends are gathered around with panic, fear, and questions on their faces. I squeeze my eyes shut again, desperate to block out the fear, and softly call to Jesse. He is there in the heartbeat of healing I'm struggling to hold onto now.

He grabs my hand, and I quickly tell him how imperative it is to remove the negativity surrounding us. I don't need to hear people questioning whether she will live or die. I need them to believe she will be fine. I fight to slip back into the ether, struggling to block out the voices and concentrate on the Love, Light, and energy that are flowing to my girl.

I rub my hands together again.

Only when I feel the pressure in my chest release do I take a deep breath and fully open my eyes.

"They're done," I announce to no one and everyone. "It worked," I state with certainty. I stand up and move back toward Jessica's room in time to see the doctors and nurses emerging.

Joan grabs my hand. "It worked," she tells me in her beautiful accent. "She is stabilizing."

"I know. Thank you." I squeeze her hand before pushing through the door and into the room to be by Jessica's side.

She doesn't look much different to me, but it's difficult to miss the tube they have inserted into the left side of her head. I gently stroke her hair and kiss her sweet face. "You are healing," I whisper to her one more time.

ADAGIO

No one else will ever know the strength of my love for you. After all, you're the only one who knows what my heart sounds like from the inside.

Kristen Proby

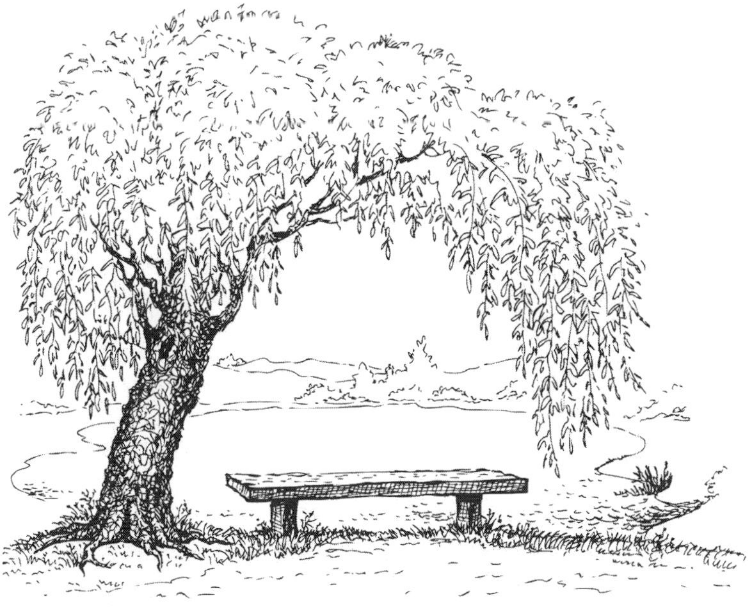

CHAPTER EIGHT

Leave Your Fear in the Fray

Jesse follows me into the room and joins me at the side of the bed. "Hey, honey," he whispers while placing his hand on the small of my back.

"Don't worry about being too quiet," I tell him. "I hope she can hear us. Talk to her."

"Hey, Jess." He touches her leg gently. "It's Dad."

"Do you think she *can* hear us?" I ask, leaning into him.

"I hope so."

As he puts his arm around me, a wave of exhaustion crashes into me so forcefully I have to grab the rail of the bed to steady myself.

"Honey?" Jesse's arm tightens around me, and he guides me to my chair-bed. He seats me on the edge and squats down in front of me. "Are you okay?"

I shake my head. "I'm so glad you're here. Nothing makes sense."

"Do you remember what happened?" He gently lifts my chin until my eyes meet his. He must think I'm close to losing my grip on reality.

I reply quickly, desperate to show him I'm coherent. "I'm well aware of what happened to Jessica. I know why we're here. I just don't remember what happened this morning. What is going on?"

It's no use. I'm able to hear the hysteria creeping into my voice, and I close my eyes again, hoping to block out the machines and monitors. I need to ground myself and find my center. *What is that quote about peace that hangs on our refrigerator at home?*

"Why don't you lie down for a minute?" Jesse suggests. "I'll stay with Jess."

I sigh and nod and then scoot back in my chair to curl up with the blanket and pillow the hospital has provided. I try to slow my breathing again, searching for the light that filled me such a short time ago.

My memory of the saying on our refrigerator surfaces:

> *Peace. It does not mean to be in a place where there is no noise, trouble, or hard work. It means to be in the midst of those things and still be calm in your heart.*

If only.

I breathe.

I am startled from my thoughts by my phone vibrating with a text alert. I grab it from the nightstand and see a message from Barb:

Jolene, what are the visiting hours? I'd like to come to the hospital to see you and Jessica.

I send a quick response. Hoping to lose myself in the mundane act of checking email and Facebook, I'm stunned by what greets me and sit up again. Dozens of emails and messages fill my inbox and Facebook wall.

... lighting candles now

... straight to our knees to pray

... inviting the bell to ring

... sending love from Oklahoma... from New York... from Las Vegas... from Portland... from Canada... from South Africa

... friend in Australia lighting candles

... told everyone in my teleconference at work this morning; people praying in Sweden, Germany, Japan, Spain

... Jane asked the school to pray for Jessica this morning

... spoke to the pastor; all 16 services at Bayside will be praying for Jessica this weekend

I am humbled by all the love and prayers that are being showered upon Jessica. Upon me. With every message I read, the circle expands, and at its center is our little girl, being showered with love.

She will be fine.

This much love and light can only lift her up for healing. In no time, I've found my center again.

A soft knock at the door pulls me back to reality. Kari is standing there with a soda and some food. I nod at her to come in.

"I'm sure you haven't eaten." She sets the food down next to my purse on the nightstand.

"Thank you. I think the Internet is saving my sanity." I give her my phone, sharing the messages that are coming in on my Facebook page faster than I can respond. She sits on the edge of the chair next to me, and tears glisten in her eyes as she reads through the messages.

We both jump as one of the IVs begins to sing its shrill melody.

"I feel like I'm living in an episode of *House*." We watch as Erik slides in, works his magic to calm the IV, checks in with the computerized sentry, and slips back out. "Minus the Vicodin and commercial breaks, of course."

Kari's usually infectious laugh has a softer quality now, which matches the quiet hum of the PICU. "I think I've only seen one or two episodes of that show."

"Dr. House is addicted to Vicodin. When the doctors do their rounds here, it reminds me of the show. They are so serious . . . except the doctor with the goatee, who even looks like House if I squint a little. He adds a bit of dark humor to ease the tension."

"Well, he's probably aware of how intently you are listening."

"You're right, though I'm not sure why I bother to listen." I pick at the threads on the scratchy hospital blanket. "They talked to us before and after the procedure this morning, but I don't remember anything they said."

"I overheard a little bit. Jessica's ICP was elevated, and they were having difficulty stabilizing it."

"ICP?" Now she's confused me.

"Intracranial pressure. Her brain is swelling from the impact, and it is causing the ICP to go up."

I swallow hard and nod at her to continue.

She takes my hand and squeezes gently. "The doctors said that the basic functions needed for survival could be compromised and that Jessica has an uncal herniation."

I rub my eyes and release a prayer of gratitude into The Universe for whatever inspired my dearest friend to become a physical therapist for children nearly twenty years ago. "Thank you for being here. I don't remember hearing the doctors say that. What is that?"

Kari suddenly seems to be possessed by Joan, the neurosurgery nurse practitioner, as she starts saying big words that I can't comprehend. I wave at her. "I'll Google it."

"Basically, when Jessica got struck, it caused a herniation that is pushing on her brainstem. The increased ICP adds to that complication, as it can restrict blood flow. That's why her basic functions could be compromised." She squeezes my hand again as I focus on Jesse, who is still standing quietly by Jessica's side.

"So, then, what was all of the commotion? I lost the entire morning."

"I came straight here after dropping Hannah off at daycare. When I arrived, Erik had taken charge and was attentively keeping track of each monitor. I could tell he was stressed and the situation was urgent. He was saying the team would be up, and they arrived a few minutes later."

I'm watching her closely now, as she fills in details I feel I should already know. As Jessica's mother, this should be my story to tell.

Kari's eyes search the nurse's area, as mine did earlier. "That doctor there…" She points discreetly. "I think that's Dr. Evans. She wanted the nail polish removed from one of Jess's toenails, and I couldn't hear much except Erik saying, 'This is why I needed you guys to get up here. We can't get the ICP stable.'"

I lift the lid of the container from the cafeteria but close it quickly.

Food seems impossible, so I grab the soda and take a sip. "I don't remember seeing her."

"Well, it was the other doctor—"

"Dr. Harlan." I set the drink down and close my eyes, hoping the room will right itself.

"Yes, Dr. Harlan. He went into the room to speak to you, but you were on the phone."

"I was trying to get Jesse here." I exhale slowly, reliving the panic.

"I know, honey. I didn't hear what the doctor was saying to you, but when Jesse finally got here and pulled you out of the room, he told me what the doctor said."

It's no easier to repeat the words for her now that Jessica is stable than it was to say them to Jesse when things were falling apart. I whisper, "He said if people were going to come, they needed to come right then."

"Right." She takes my hand and squeezes tight. It's exactly what I need to keep me grounded. "That's when I started texting people to start a prayer chain, asking for prayers for her survival and for the doctors to use their knowledge to make the best decisions regarding medical intervention for her."

The hairs on my arm rise, and I shake off the chill running down my spine as the realization hits me. "That's what I was meditating on at the same moment." I inch even closer to her on the small chair and lay my head on her shoulder. Kari continues her report.

"As more people started arriving, I took them down to the family area to try to explain what I knew. When we all came back to the hallway here, the doctors had decided to place a shunt to relieve the ICP."

"That's the new tube on the left side of her head?"

"If it wasn't there this morning, then yes. That's the shunt. It will help drain the fluid so the pressure on her brain can be decreased."

I look into the hall outside the room and see family and friends still gathered around, speaking to one another quietly.

"I should go out and talk to everyone, but even after all you've told me, what am I supposed to say?"

Kari finally releases her grip on me and stands up. "You don't need to worry about them right now. Get some rest. I'll go talk to them."

Too exhausted to protest, I thank her and lie back down. "I love you, K."

"I love you, too." She turns to go, but a thought strikes me, and I stop her.

"Kare?"

"Yeah."

"So, Erik? He's basically my hero?"

"He saved Jessica's life."

She says this so seriously, and the gravity of our morning once again threatens to take me down.

Somehow I keep breathing.

CHAPTER NINE

I Thought of Just Your Face

I'm supposed to be resting, but whenever I close my eyes, the most painful images no parent should ever have to see are in the forefront of my mind. When I open my eyes, I am overwhelmed by everything I don't understand in this hospital room.

Trying to escape to the comfort of family and friends clustered in the hallway leaves me feeling even more uneasy and scattered. Taking refuge in the bathroom down the hall only results in my breaking down when I suddenly hit the wall of this reality: My little Mini-Me is lying in the best PICU in our region, fighting for her life.

So I sit, hour after hour, watching Jessica and rubbing my hands together slowly while I play the words in my head over and over again. *You are healing. You will be fine.*

Every time I ask if Jessica is doing better or if she's going to be okay, the nurses avoid meeting my eyes or giving me a straight answer. They tell me it's too soon to know anything and we will probably move to the "real" PICU at some point, as where we are now is in the overflow wing. I'm learning that time moves very differently in the hospital than it does in the real world, so when "at some point" will occur is anyone's guess. I should probably find solace in a planned move, however, figuring they wouldn't plan to move her if they didn't think she'd survive.

I try to listen in whenever the doctors are around. While I don't understand a great majority of the medical speak, I find that I do love the way they talk about Jessica's treatment and the little things they do for her physically. They talk about it in terms of what she likes. She wasn't tolerating one medication at a high dose but didn't respond well when they tried to cut it off completely, so Dr. Harlan said she is getting "just a whiff" of it and "she likes that."

It is comforting in a strange sort of way. Not only is their medical expertise apparent, but the doctors and nurses are paying attention to how Jessica tolerates being moved into a certain position or how the smallest dose of a given medication affects her. They speak of her as a person, not just a patient, and I am grateful for this attention to detail.

I imagine they are motivated by the very nature of their jobs to bring Jessica back. But if they can see her as more than a patient, if they connect with her as the sweet and amazing child that we love so much, then I hope it adds an extra level of determination to their motivation.

The doctor who reminds me of Dr. House, whose name I've learned is Dr. Pretzlaff, is able to tell me that we are still on a minute-to-minute watch and Jessica's condition is still very critical. The situation continues to be life and death.

Each of the doctors and nurses share bits and pieces of the medical information with me, using terms like *uncal herniation*, *midline shift*, *posturing*, and *neurological assessment*. I try to understand as much as I can, but their words have no value, as I lack the education to determine which are positive references, which are negative, and which simply are. I consider my questions carefully, not wanting to interfere with their focus on Jessica and also being honest with myself about how much more information I can process right now.

Jessica has been heavily sedated and is medically paralyzed. I understand that the doctors want to take her off the paralytics so they will be able to test her responses, but what I don't understand completely are her numbers. It's a cruel joke that they've put someone with an affinity for numbers in a room with a monitor that shows half a dozen stats I can't seem to decipher. I know they tell at a glance where Jessica stands, and it's frustrating that I don't understand what they mean. What I wouldn't give for a cheat sheet to help me unlock the secret code.

Some of the readings are obvious. I'm guessing HR is heart rate, fairly confident that BP is blood pressure, and pretty sure that ICP is the intracranial pressure that Kari told me about. But what are CVP and CPP?

I study the monitor throughout the day, willing it to release its inner secrets and magic to me. I see the levels rise and fall, but the key to what it means for Jessica's survival remains elusive.

Kari is back from a coffee run and checks in with me again. We sit in silence, holding hands, as I remain mesmerized by the glow of the monitors.

"They are monitoring everything right now," Kari says softly. "Her blood pressure, her heart rate, the swelling in her brain, her temperature..."

I sigh, so grateful for Kari, who, after twenty-five years of friendship, is more sister than friend. "Which one tells me she is in there and that she's going to be okay?"

"Oh, honey." She squeezes my hand again.

"I know." I rub my eyes with my free hand. "She will be fine."

Friday becomes Saturday, and sleep continues to evade me. It's 4:00 a.m., and I am still so amped up on adrenaline that I can't sit and do nothing. So I am composing the email I told Melissa I would send to the dance families. I hope it will help me collect my thoughts and process everything that has been thrown at us.

Hello, families,

We could really use any good energy, thoughts, or prayers that you can send our way. As Jessica was preparing her horse for her riding lesson on Thursday, another horse unexpectedly ran into the area she was in and attempted to kick her horse, who moved out of the way, leaving Jessica unprotected.

This all occurred in a split second and is truly a freak accident. We do not blame anyone for it and believe it was unavoidable.

We were taken immediately—really incredible response time from South Placer County Fire—to Sutter Roseville Medical Center, where she was in surgery for about three and a half hours.

She had part of her skull removed, as part of it was crushed, and her brain needs a place to go when it begins swelling.

She was in a coma when we got to the hospital, but post-surgery she was somewhat awake and responsive. Once they were able to get her stable, we were transferred to the PICU at UC Davis Children's Hospital.

Once we got to UCD, they needed to get control of the pressure that was building in her head, and they need to keep stimulation to the brain to a minimum, so they have medically induced a coma. Things were very scary and at the most critical between 1:00 a.m. and 10:00 a.m. yesterday morning. They told us "everyone who should be here, needs to get here," and they ended up inserting a drain into the left side of her head.

Thankfully, she responded well to the procedure, and she has been fairly stable since.

The next day or two are the most critical, and we are currently in a wait-and-see status for the next 48–72 hours. We are probably looking at a 2–3 week hospital stay.

I am overwhelmed at the severity of the information I am sharing with these families, with whom I have spent dozens of hours every week for the past several years. I remind myself these are the details I would want to hear if it were a member of their family. I just don't want the situation to sound as serious as it sounds.

I throw in the address for the hospital, share what she can and cannot have (no latex or flowers but yes to stuffed animals and Mylar balloons), ask for cards and pictures from her buddies, and tell them we welcome visitors, if they are called to visit. I add contact information for Jesse and me and search for something that will ease the tension of such a heavy email.

I will try to keep everyone as informed as I can. Hug all those girls tight, and good luck at competition this weekend. Give them a "Go, girls!" for me, and we look forward to hearing all about it in a month or so.

I hit Send and then sit back and stare at the monitors.

Before I can blink, morning rounds are starting. I float to Jessica's side again, trying to take in bits and pieces of her, looking for movement or any sign that she is coming back to me, besides my own unwavering thoughts that *she will be fine.*

The bruising around her right eye is more apparent, darkening to various shades of blue and purple. Her eyes glisten from the ointment the nurses put in every few hours to keep them from drying out. Her lips are dry and cracked, and I think about grabbing the Vaseline I've seen the nurses use for this purpose, but I'm not sure where they keep it and don't want to start poking around.

The doctors make their way toward Jessica's room, and I prop the door open and listen to their morning report. They start with the easily understandable part... her name, her age, and her injury... but quickly slide into the medical talk, and I'm lost. They rattle off her medications and the rate at which she is receiving each before relaying the plan to lower the paralytic and try to get into the other PICU wing by the end of the day.

The nursing shift changes, and the new nurse comes in, adjusts the IVs, records Jessica's vital signs, and checks in with the computer sentry.

This is pretty much the order for the day. Nurses and doctors coming in and out, checking Jessica's numbers and adjusting her IVs. While things don't feel as frantic and chaotic as they did yesterday, I once again pick up on the fact that something is not quite right. I can't bear the thought of what could be going wrong or hearing more bad news, so I sit, numb, watching the medical staff work their magic hour after hour.

By the end of the day, I have a clearer picture of what has occurred. Piecing together the easy parts of the conversations, I begin to understand that they tried to take Jessica off the paralytic this morning in order to perform the neurological assessments and test her responses, but Jessica didn't like it. The changes caused her blood pressure to rise, which, in turn, raised the pressure in her brain, so the doctors and nurses spent the rest of the day trying to correct the error.

Evening has fallen, and Jessica is stable again. As much as I want her to wake up and as curious as I am about the results of their assessments (especially if it tells us when she will wake up completely from her coma), I really just want them to leave her alone. I want her to have a chance to rest, to recover more and gain some strength before they start messing with things again.

For now, it seems as though they agree, and I try to relax a bit, sitting and talking quietly with my niece, Amanda, who arrived this afternoon.

The PICU takes on an ethereal feel as the hour grows late and the family and friends of all the patients begin to break away, one by one, heading for the safety of familiar beds and the arms of their loved ones. Even Jesse left, if reluctantly, to pick up Jocelyn and take her home to get her to bed at a decent hour.

Exhaustion is creeping into my bones, but I continue to put off lying down to rest, because the night shift nurses keep telling us we will be moving any minute now. As the last woman standing, Amanda helps me pack up the care items that have been delivered today. We bunch all of the balloons together, and the nurses give us a bag in which to transport the many cards, pictures, stuffed animals, and little altar items.

After a lot of hurry-up-and-wait, we finally make our way around the corner and down the hall to set up shop in Bed Six. They tell us this will be Jess's permanent room until she is up and ready to transfer to our HMO's hospital for rehabilitation. I hug Amanda goodbye and text Jesse to tell him she is heading to the house. She plans to stay with us for a couple of days, until we have more answers about Jessica's condition.

The nurses are still getting Jessica settled and watching the monitors closely to see how she tolerated the move, but we've been here for about half an hour, and things are looking stable. In fact, she likes this space, I think. They say her readings look a smidge better than they did before the move.

The night nurse and her trainee are young, cute, and approachable. Just the kind of young women Jessica naturally gravitates toward. As they move about, I'm able to ask them questions about what they're doing.

While changing out the lines to Jessica's IVs, they explain to me that "spaghetti" is a term for all of the lines, tubes, and wires just hanging around in a mess. These women work together to get the lines changed over and the spaghetti cleaned up.

They let me in on the inner secrets of the monitors and what I should be looking for. Most of it goes over my head again, but they make sure to point out the important stats to watch. The blood pressure (BP), intracranial pressure (ICP), and cerebral profusion pressure (CPP) give the doctors a picture of the pressure that is in Jessica's head.

They further explain what happened when the doctors tried to reduce the paralytic earlier in the day. It caused Jessica's BP to rise, which is what makes the ICP and CPP go up. It took all day for them to regain control of those levels, but they assure me things are looking stable now. So much so that they are getting ready to give her a bath and change her bed linens.

They bring in piles of new linens, a bath bin, towels, and soap and begin removing things from Jessica's bed. They strip the blanket and Jessica's hospital gown and begin the dance of bathing her. One washes her with a soaped-up washcloth, while the other follows with a clean washcloth and towel. They work quickly, making sure Jessica doesn't stay too wet in one place for too long.

Watching this ritual feels powerful on some level. Seeing Jessica with nothing covering her but wires and tubes is difficult. But being able to see her beautiful body in all its glory and believe that it is healing and still strong is a beautiful thing.

As the nurses move in a circle around her bed, I find myself absentmindedly rubbing my hands together while creating a silly little rhyme.

We are the circle;

She is our center.

As we move in, we release the pressure.

The energy is released into The Universe,

Neutralized before making things worse.

One clear voice, let this be heard.

The nurses finish getting Jessica dried and redressed and finally sit down at the computer to update their charts.

"Her numbers are still improving," the training nurse comments as she types stats into the computer. "She likes this room. I think she's happy here."

I finally pull out the chair-bed and curl up under the blanket while thinking that it's obvious Jessica likes our new home.

We are in the ocean.

The décor in this section of the PICU is the ocean. There is a whale tail on the wall behind the nurses' station and dolphins and mermaids on the walls leading to her door. Fish and waves adorn the surrounding walls. There are cliffs and mountains on the walls of Jessica's room, which means the bed is in the part of the ocean leading up to the shore.

Jessica is buoyed here by the sea.

As I drift off to sleep, visions of Jessica on the deck of the Princess Monterey last year fill my head. To celebrate Jessica's birthday in March, we surprised her with a trip to Monterey for sight-seeing and whale watching. Jessica was enamored with the entire experience, but being on the boat was definitely the highlight.

We saw whales and dolphins, a sea turtle, sea birds, a jellyfish, and sea lions. It was the perfect trip.

In one of my favorite pictures of her, the ocean and the rail of the boat are in the background. She is wearing her pink jacket and her glasses. As her hair blows in the sea spray, she looks over her shoulder at me, an excited smile on her face.

It was the best day with her. That day.

CHAPTER TEN

All Your Grace and Style

The morning rounds have already started, and they'll be by to check on Jessica in a few minutes. Lying here, watching the doctors talk in the hallway, I wipe the sleep from my eyes and try to hold onto my dream.

Just a few short days ago while lying in the dirt next to Jessica, I told her she was exactly where she needed to be. That she should allow Mother Earth to reach up and comfort her. That the Angels were swooping down, protecting her. And I told her, "Grandpa is here. He is not going to let anything happen to you. Your Grandpa is here."

Last night, I dreamt that my dad rode in on Katie, Jessica's horse from the barn. Katie walked right through the double doors of Jessica's small hospital room, and my dad looked down on his granddaughter with the same love he shone on her the day she was born.

When the doctors approach Jessica's room, I stand just outside her door, listening to the script that is becoming more familiar, even if I don't understand the majority of it. The rounds have a more positive feel to them. No new information is being shared, and nothing major has changed, but that, in and of itself, can be seen as a good thing. We have been in the new room for six or seven hours, and Jessica's numbers remain stable. As the doctors wind down their report of Jessica's overnight status, I take the rare opportunity to involve myself in the rounds, asking Dr. Pretzlaff if things are better than they were yesterday.

"You're trying to get more than I have to give you." He answers in the way that I have come to understand is the "real picture" these doctors want to paint. However, I notice that the stress of the previous day is not in his face. His features are relaxed, and his blue eyes sparkle rather than darken.

Things feel different.

Couple this little bit of not-much news with the dream I had last night, and a fire is lit in my heart. A fire of hope that the Angels' words will come true. A fire of certainty that Jessica will be fine.

With each hour that passes, more visitors come to see Jessica and to check on me. Most of Jesse's family live in another city, state, or country, but various members of my family stop by. There are visits from dance friends and Kari's family, who are like a second family to me. Becky and Steve come by again, as well as a woman who gave Jessica piano lessons the previous year. She asks if she can pray for Jessica. I say, "Of course," thinking she means in church on Sunday or when she gets home. I am surprised and overwhelmed with emotion when she goes to her knees next to Jessica's hospital bed.

When visitors arrive, I often take the opportunity to check in with the nurses or doctors and get information about Jessica's latest numbers. With each hour that passes with no negative changes, the fire in my heart glows brighter. By the end of the day, I feel manic. I know my good mood is out of proportion with the fact that Jessica remains in a coma, but I am positively beaming from the fact that she remains stable.

I think some adjustments have been made to her medications here and there, or maybe the nurses are just replacing empty bags, but nothing they do causes the type of fluctuations in her numbers or the amount of stress that occurred yesterday.

She is healing. She will be fine.

"Are you ready to give me more now?" I ask Dr. Pretzlaff in the evening, trying to keep my voice light.

He smiles at me, chuckling a little bit. "I can't give you more than I have, but yes. She has remained stable all day. I believe her swelling has peaked."

I resist the urge to hug and kiss him and return to Jessica's room to study her again, searching for signs that support his thinking. It does look like her color has smoothed out. The nurses must have been busy with the IVs today, as there is no spaghetti by the machines or covering Jessica's body.

I barely notice that Dr. Pretzlaff has followed me into the room. "I'm sorry to ask you this again, but now that she is more stable, can you tell me what you remember?"

"What I remember...?" I straighten up, looking at him and then back at Jessica. Her special Thomy bear is tucked under her arm, along with a few more "stuffies," as she calls them, which were delivered as gifts. "She just looks like she's sleeping."

"I know," The doctor says softly. "But you know she's—"

"Not. Yeah, I know."

"I can come back, but it would help if you don't mind talking to me a bit longer."

"Right, right... what I remember." I follow him out of the room, softly closing the door behind us. "Can we talk right here?" I ask, looking through the window at Jessica.

"That would be fine. So, what happened? What do you remember?"

"Everything." I sigh. "I remember everything."

I remember the impatience I felt the morning of her birth, when they kept me in recovery for four hours before getting me into a room and letting me hold my brand new daughter. I remember the first song I ever sang to her and how my dearly departed dad was the only person in the room to witness that moment.

I remember the instability and uncertainty of our lives when she was a baby and a toddler. I remember finding joy in the times when she would play in the kitchen drawers or get into mischief.

I remember sharing a room with her when we moved out on our own and her acting like a rock star on the bed when my hard rock music was playing. She tore all of the blankets and pillows off the bed and threw them around.

I remember worrying about the man who came to save us from the instability and uncertainty and whether or not I could trust him with my daughter's heart.

I remember beaming at each and every interaction they had in the beginning, watching him with her and not intervening, my test of whether he would cut the snuff as a parent.

I remember preschool at Brighton and falling in love with all of her little buddies there and finding myself grateful that we still have connections with many of them.

I remember the first "official" picture we took at Tricks Gymnastics and Dance, as well as all that followed over the next seven years. I definitely remember the coaches and how much she loves them all, even long after leaving their classes.

I remember early elementary school at Brighton; her "boyfriends" Collin, Andrew, and Thomas; and her turning into a tomboy in second grade in order to hang with all of the boys.

I remember the rough transitions to public school in third grade and the move to a different district when we purchased our first house.

I remember long discussions about things that I wonder if I should have discussed with her so soon. Teaching her about her body parts early and telling her how babies were made when she asked, as well as boring stuff like money and bills. Helping her through conflicts with friends but reaching a point where I forced myself to be hands off, telling her, "You gotta handle it on your own."

I remember knowing that she is my constant star. That anything I can do for her, I will.

I remember teaching her that we will get angry at each other, but the one thing that never changes is love. I remember making her repeat that to me nearly every time we had an argument or I was angry with her.

I remember that she is not the perfect kid and I am not the perfect parent, but we are perfect for one another.

I remember playing songs for her that I thought she should hear: "Imagine" by John Lennon, "Everything Possible" by Fred Small, "I Just Love You" by Five for Fighting, and, of course, "You Gotta Be" by Des'Ree, the song I sang to her the day she was born.

I remember making her French toast three mornings ago. I remember putting dinner in the Crock-Pot, knowing she would love it because it had mushrooms and onions in it. I remember being in awe of her weird eating habits and constantly trying to work around them.

I remember the laughter and her smile, teasing back and forth, and her rolling her eyes at me. She knows how dedicated I am and always will be to her, and I know that she is one of the two greatest kids on the face of this earth, for whom I will move mountains.

I remember bitterness and anger and how it can swallow you whole. I remember love and compassion and Divine Intervention.

"Ms. Lavine?" Dr. Pretzlaff interrupts the movie playing in my head.

I am barely breathing. "What do I remember? I remember it all," I tell him as I walk to a bench in the hall. "I sit alone with her in that room, watching her 'sleep'. There is nothing to do but replay every moment of her life. I think about the impact on her of every decision I and others have made, and I feel love swirling around her, just as it has every day of her life."

"I understand." His gaze is soft and kind again, and I close my eyes before taking a deep breath and telling our story.

CHAPTER ELEVEN

Impromptu for 12 Fingers

May 6, 2010 – One Week Post-Accident

The longer we are in the hospital, the more adept I become at the steps of the dance of the PICU. I'm learning when to change partners, when to sit it out, and when to jump into the free-for-all of organized chaos on the stage.

Jessica has been "sleeping" through it all, of course. She's missed the nursing changes, the doctors' rounds, the x-rays each morning, and even the ultrasound of her brain.

The doctors ordered the scan because they suspected the veins in Jessica's head were seizing, which meant her brain would not receive adequate oxygen. The radiology tech came in and began connecting electrodes of many different colors all over Jessica's scalp.

The new activity caused Jessica's blood pressure to rise, and there went her numbers again. I updated my status on Facebook, asking people to send Jessica calming thoughts to help her blood pressure normalize. Within a few minutes, the nurses noticed that the position of her bed was contributing to the rise in her blood pressure. It was an easy fix, and the tech finished hooking up the electrodes and completed the test.

The initial report showed Jessica's veins might, in fact, be seizing, so the nurses rushed her to CT to investigate the issue further.

Thankfully, Jesse had the morning off work, so he could offer more support at the hospital. He volunteered to go down to CT so one of us would be close to Jessica. Based on past experience with radiology, we thought the scan would take an hour or two, so I agreed. I sent out another prayer request to Facebook, asking the masses to envision Jessica's veins open and pumping adequate blood to her beautiful brain, and then I rushed off to take a shower.

The soap and shampoo had barely made it down the drain before Jesse texted me to let me know the CT was done, Jessica's veins were open, and the nurses were bringing her back up. *I need to remember to ask Facebook for lottery numbers,* I thought to myself, as I dressed quickly and returned to the room.

Through it all, Jessica continued to "sleep."

She missed another bath, the changing out of her bed because of an electronics issue, a second and much less eventful ultrasound, breathing treatments, and the removal and relocation of various IVs.

During all the busywork that was performed, I held my breath, worried that Jessica would get too agitated and her numbers would go haywire again. My worries unfounded, Jessica sailed through the changes. Her ICP fell consistently, reaching the lowest level we'd seen to that point.

It's a week after the accident, and the doctors have been able to turn off the paralytic and sedative without causing Jessica's BP to rise. They warned me she might begin to experience some pain and recommended restricting visitors in order to keep the stimulation to a minimum.

This means I'm alone with Jessica more often. I sit, studying her for any twitch, flinch, or change in position she might make. I keep an inventory of the stages of her bruises and swelling. Today, the swelling in her right eye looks a little less severe. Melissa described it as really pretty stage makeup. To add to the stage effect, even though Jessica's hair has been shaved on both sides, she has a mass of curls in the middle that reminds me of *So You Think You Can Dance* choreographer Sonya Tayeh.

Suddenly I'm lost in the memory of the swirls of one of Jessica's dance costumes from the competition year, a lightly tie-dyed orange dress that flowed and twirled with each move of the number Melissa titled "The Flower Dance." The piano notes for that dance seem to fill the air, and all I see is Jessica swirling around the stage.

I'm sure I should be paying more attention to what she's saying. I can't seem to look away.

Jesse and I are sitting in a tiny office off the PICU for a meeting with the doctor, hoping to learn how Jessica is doing.

The doctor, a lovely woman named Stephanie Mateev, has pulled up Jessica's CT films on the computer. The black-and-white images capture my attention. In opposition to the way I seemed to hear only the good information in our meeting with Dr. Bosco a week earlier, all I can hear and see now is the devastation before me.

The pictures glow side by side, one taken in the emergency room directly after the accident and the other taken three days ago after the ultrasound.

They show my brilliant, funny, sweet, kind baby girl's precious brain shifted in her skull. The ER CT shows the pieces of broken bone that were removed in surgery, along with a two- to three centimeter section of her brain above her right ear.

I understand little of what Dr. Mateev is saying. I hear only the worst parts: Left-side paralysis. Blindness. Deafness. Seizures. Pneumonia. Death.

I can't look away.

"... the *good news* is ..."

Finally tearing my eyes away from the computer screen, I meet Dr. Mateev's pointed gaze. "The good news is we are out of life-and-death danger as a result of the injury. While the other complications I've outlined are possible, it is highly unlikely Jessica will die from the injury itself. We are out of the woods in that regard."

Jesse and I look at each other. I see my conflict mirrored in his beautiful blue eyes. She's no longer in danger, except that she is?

"It could be up to two years," Dr. Mateev continues, "for your daughter to be back to herself."

I look at the screen again. "But that's possible?"

"Anything is," she says softly. "The possibilities I've laid out for you, though difficult to hear, are very possible. Realistic, even. If I don't give you the worst-case scenario, you will be unprepared for what's to come. I can't provide false hope and say she will recover. It's only been a week. We don't know that, but yes. Anything is possible."

I close my eyes and breathe. *False hope? Is there such a thing? Isn't it just hope? If anything can happen, if they can't be sure one way or the other, then why can't the best happen? Why shouldn't I continue to hope for that?*

I turn to Jesse and state with certainty, "She will be fine."

"But honey . . . ," he says gently, glancing at the doctor.

"It's only been a week! I won't give up on her. Knowing she will survive is the best news we've received since the accident. I will sit in that chair in this hospital for as long as it takes if it means my baby girl is coming back to me. So, what happens next?"

My question is soon answered by a flurry of hospital activity that all starts to run together. After the doctors turned off the paralytic and lowered the sedative dose, there seemed to be something new every minute.

Now the minor occurrences are the constant checking and removal of IVs (she's down to two!) and the almost constant review of her vitals on the monitor and her reflexes. They've removed her catheter, and she has started eliminating normally again. The swelling is visibly decreased, and even though she is still on the ventilator, we've been told she's breathing on her own.

Jessica has also begun "storming," which is the term used when the brain tries to re-fire and rewire itself. I'm sure this process presents itself differently in each patient, but for Jessica it comes with an increase in her heart rate and blood pressure, accompanied by fever, shaking, and agitation. It is difficult to watch, because the doctors discourage even gentle touching during the rewiring process. What we think of as a gentle and reassuring touch can be wired as pain right now.

But the storming seems to be working. Jessica continues to make bigger movements with her body. Instead of shaking and trembling, she is moving her legs up and down. She moves her arms around and even rolls her shoulders. It's almost as if her skin is a suit she is shrugging into, trying to get comfortable again.

At this point, my biggest frustration comes from trying to convince the doctors that some of the movements Jessica makes seem to hold great meaning.

When Melissa came to visit, the minute she walked through the door, Jessica's left arm came up and her hand began clenching, as if she was reaching for Melissa. "Must . . . reach . . . dance . . . coach."

Doctor's response: "Coincidence."

Or the time she moved her arms up during a breathing treatment, as if to push the therapist away?

"Reflexive."

The kicker was when the sun was going down, and I was looking at a card her friend Anna made for her. Jessica and Anna share a love of *Percy Jackson and the Olympians* books, which center around the Greek gods. Anna wrote in her card, "Get well soon, Daughter of Apollo."

My niece, Amanda, was visiting again and needed a refresher course to know which god Apollo was. So I read to her from Wikipedia.

Apollo has been recognized as a god of light and the sun; truth and prophecy; archery; medicine, healing and plague; music, poetry and the arts.

As I read out loud, the sun was setting and hit Jessica in the face. She turned away and tried to bring her hands up, as if to cover her face.

To me, this demonstrated intent and purpose: "The sun is in my eyes; please remove it now."

The doctor's interpretation? "Spontaneous stimulation and her neurons re-firing."

I'm going to take *my* explanation to bed with me tonight to keep me warm. She is moving. She is fighting to get back to us.

CHAPTER TWELVE

When You Find You

"Good morning, Ms. Lavine."

It's Dr. Natale this time. Eleven days in, and I still haven't gotten everyone's roles straight, but at least I'm starting to learn their names.

"Jolene, please." I smile at her from the side of Jessica's bed, where I've been talking and singing to her softly as she seems to wake up more.

"We have a couple of things to do this morning. We're going to take Jessica off the vent and remove her drain." She says this casually as she examines Jessica and checks the ever-present monitor. I simply stare at her, unsure how to react.

"She's ready. Her ICP and her oxygen levels have remained stable. We'll remove the drain and keep a close watch on her ICP. The breathing tube will be replaced with an oxygen mask. If her levels continue to do well, we'll replace the mask with a nasal cannula. The O2 flow will be decreased until she is breathing on her own."

Dr. Natale is barely done with her assessment and explanations when a team of people descend on the room. I move toward the end of the bed to allow them access to Jessica. This is where being on visitor restriction is a major drawback. I don't have time to process what's going to happen before they are pulling the tube from Jessica's throat, and my knees buckle.

"Jolene!" Dr. Natale reaches out to steady me, and I grab the side of the bed to catch my balance.

Before my own heart rate can return to normal, the doctors fit an oxygen mask over Jessica's face and begin to remove the drain on the left side of her head.

Overwhelmed by emotion, I let go of the side of the bed and step back so I can sit down on a chair.

"It's going to be okay." Dr. Natale kneels down and places her hands on my knees. "She's ready for this. We wouldn't do anything that would endanger her life."

"I know." I fight through the lump in my throat. "It's just... that's the drain that saved her life. Without it, there would have been no miracle. We would be without Jessica." I shake my head and wipe at the tears that have escaped. "I'm sorry."

"Don't be. I understand." She pats my knees gently before standing to join the team as they leave the room, taking the ventilator with them.

With the big machine out of the way, I'm able to get even closer to Jessica's head than before. I take full advantage and pull my chair up to the head of her bed, where I continue to talk and sing to my sweet girl.

"You are healing, strong girl. Just come back to me."

"Happy Mother's Day, honey." Jesse and Jocelyn have arrived for the day.

"Thank you. I got a nice present today," I tell Jesse while hugging Jocelyn to me.

"Oh?" Jesse leans down to kiss me and then leans over to say hello to Jessica. "Oh!" He gestures toward the empty space where the ventilator once sat.

"Yep. They removed the breathing tube this morning. She was on an oxygen mask for a couple of hours, but they changed her to the nose prongs a bit ago. They think they'll be able to turn off the oxygen within a few hours."

"And she's doing okay?" He makes his way over to look at the monitor and nods at what he sees there.

"Yeah, and that's not all. They also removed the drain." I point to her head.

"Oh, good."

"Yeah, poor Dr. Natale. She nearly had to catch me. It all happened so fast. I didn't expect to react so emotionally. I almost fainted."

"Oh, baby." He comes over to rub my shoulders, and I grab his hand and squeeze. "Do you want to get some air? Spend some time with Joce?"

"Yeah, I better take her out of here, at least. We'll be back in a bit." I grab some cash from my purse, scoop up my Littlest Bean, and head out the door.

I stop by the coffee kiosk before taking Jocelyn outside to let her burn off some energy. As she plays on the steps in front of the hospital entrance, going up and down before walking the full length of each level, I try to memorize every bit of her.

Not only have I lost the joy of my daily routine with Jessica, but I haven't been able to see much of Jocelyn. I'm without both of my girls. It makes my heart ache in a way I have to box up and compartmentalize, only taking it out to examine in bits and pieces.

A familiar buzz pulls me from my thoughts, and I fish my phone out of my pocket.

Honey, the doctors need to talk to both of us.

I stand quickly and grab Jocelyn, running to the elevators. *I knew I shouldn't have left.* I punch the UP button over and over again until the car arrives, and I rush in. I set Jocelyn down and try to concentrate on her joy at holding onto the handrails and jumping up and down on the ride.

We finally make it to the seventh floor, and I take Jocelyn's little hand to let her skip along with me as I hurry to the door of the PICU and push the doorbell. Once admitted, I pull the door open. Just as I am beginning to sprint to our room at the end of the hall,

I see Jesse at the nurse's station with Dr. Natale and a woman with short blond hair.

"What's wrong?" I ask, slowing down but not stopping. I inch past them, anxious to reach Jessica's room.

"Nothing. Nothing is wrong." Jesse picks up Jocelyn and grabs my hand, pulling me closer to them. "They want to talk to us about transferring Jessica to our HMO hospital."

"What? Why?"

"Ms. Lavine, my name is Jodie, and I'm one of the discharge planners here. Fortunately, Jessica's condition has progressed to the point that she is no longer in need of intensive care. This means she can be transferred to the regular pediatric floor."

"Okay, but why do we have to leave here? I'd rather keep her here. You are the best children's hospital."

"Thank you for that. Unfortunately, because your HMO has a pediatric floor—"

"But—" Before I can voice any further objections, Jesse squeezes my hand.

"Honey, let's just listen for a minute. This is actually good news."

"Jesse is right," Dr. Natale confirms. "With the removal of the breathing tube and the ICP drain this morning, Jessica's medical support right now is minimal. She is no longer on any continuous IVs, and her medications can be given to her through her NG tube. She is no longer in critical condition, so your HMO wants her."

I try to keep my voice level. "But she's not *better*. All the things they've been telling us... responding to yes-or-no questions, talking, any kind of response. She's not doing that yet."

"I know it's difficult, Ms. Lavine," Jodie explains, "but your insurance plan does not cover a pediatric stay in another hospital when they have one available."

"Can we pay privately, then?" I am desperate not to leave these people who know my daughter, who saved my daughter's life.

"That would be cost prohibitive," she states simply, and the three of them look at me expectantly.

"There's nothing we can do to stay here?" I'm not surprised or ashamed to hear the pleading in my voice.

"I'm sorry. We'll let you know when we have more specifics." Dr. Natale and Jodie take a few steps back, indicating there is nothing more to be said. I try my best to storm off in a huff but achieve nothing more than a dejected shuffle the length of the hall to Jessica's room.

I'm sure this is supposed to be good news, but I'm not there yet. I'm just not there.

CHAPTER THIRTEEN

I Need a Second Opinion

The move to our HMO hospital went as smoothly as you might expect. I choked up when I realized we were walking out of the UC Davis Children's Hospital PICU for good. In such a short time, I'd grown to love the doctors and nurses so much. They cared for my child. They saved her life! I was in tears as we waved our goodbyes and headed to the elevator.

Once we were outside, though, it was a joy to see the sun shine on Jessica's face for the first time in twelve days, if only for the brief moment between the hospital and the ambulance. It helped me focus on the future, when she will be up and about and soaking in the sunshine again.

The ambulance delivered us to the new hospital, and we were routed to the PICU here. After settling in, we had an afternoon of meetings with the nurses, ICU doctor, neurosurgeon, therapists, and admissions. We discussed Jessica's case, shared our evaluations and opinions on her progress, and began taking over some of Jessica's daily routine, such as the suctioning of her secretions and her oral care.

At this point, I feel like I'm in a movie. Or maybe a television series. Everything is running together. Providing updates to everyone feels overwhelming. I could give a day-by-day, blow-by-blow report of every procedure done, movement made, meeting attended, infection cleared, x-ray taken . . . but writing an update often feels as long and tedious as living through the minutiae.

What I really want to move past is *this hospital.* The doctors are great at giving us basic information . . . it will take four to six weeks for the swelling in Jess's head to completely dissipate and three to six months before her skull can be repaired. But information like when she will start responding to us, walking, or talking . . . not so much. They hedge their bets and provide "realistic" assessments, and even when Jessica responds according to their request, they are only haltingly hopeful.

Instead of waiting for the nurses to arrive, Jesse and I have been taking the initiative to change Jessica, make her more comfortable, or manage her AFOs. AFOs are ankle foot orthotics, big, clunky splints Jessica wears for two-hour intervals in order to prevent foot-drop.

We are being more forward about her medications, and I can see the resentment in the nurses' eyes when I've done something they consider to be their job, but I can't be bothered to care. They are treating Jessica like a number, a job, or a set of routines to check off their schedule before punching out for the day. They have succeeded in making an already stressful situation completely overwhelming and unbearable.

That's exactly what I'm telling them during a family meeting when the doctor from the pediatric floor gently interrupts me. "I'm sorry you feel that way, Ms. Lavine. We do care about your daughter's progress, but there is only so much we can do."

"I don't understand that! I don't even feel like everyone is on the same page." Jesse holds his hand up in an attempt to slow my momentum and pulls in closer to the conference table. I snatch up the pen that sits on the pad of paper in front of me and begin flicking it in circles with my right hand, trying to calm my nerves. Jesse really should control this conversation. I am already emotional and volatile enough where my children are concerned. Combine that with a severe lack of sleep, my questionable eating habits over the past six weeks, and the fact that I am on the tail end of my period, and I am ready to bring this place to the ground.

Instead, I sit and spin my pen, glaring at the doctors on the other side of the conference table. They include a pediatric doctor, the neurosurgeon, a physical therapist, the care coordinator, a social worker, and a discharge planner. With the exception of Nicole, the physical therapist, who has been the only bright light in our stay here, I haven't received a straight answer about Jessica's medical needs or recovery from any of them. It's no wonder we're having a hard time getting on the same page.

"I think we just need to have an understanding of what is happening." Jesse makes the statement calmly and diplomatically while I attempt to keep my huffing to a minimum.

The peds doctor glances at the discharge planner and the social worker before addressing Jesse directly. "Well . . . what is happening with what?"

I drop the pen and slam my hand on the table. Jesse grabs it and says, "Maybe we should take a break."

I shake off his hand and put mine on the table again, gripping the edge tightly. "I'm fine, I'm fine, I'm fine. I'm fine. I just . . . I don't believe this. Why don't we start at the beginning? Let's just have a review of what is going on with Jessica right now. Then maybe you can tell us where we go from here."

I tap my fingers on the table while the doctors and therapists review their notes. The neurosurgeon clears his throat before speaking. "That is a great idea, Ms. Lavine. Let's start with the basics. Jessica is on minimal medical intervention right now. Her Glasgow Coma Scale score rose from a nine to an eleven this morning when she wiggled her toes for the pediatric team when they did their rounds."

Some of the anger drains out of me in an instant. "It did? Why weren't we told that?"

The pediatric physician responds. "I didn't want to speak out of turn or get your hopes up too much."

"Get my hopes up?" I shake my head in an attempt to shake away the tears that are threatening to rise up. I want to hold on to my anger just a bit longer in order to make it through this meeting. "I could tell it meant something when it happened! You asked her to wiggle her toes, and she did! I asked you if that meant anything! Why didn't you tell me?"

"I'm sorry; it just isn't a sure sign that she will fully recover. It simply raised her GCS."

I stare at him and will my body to stop shaking.

The Glasgow Coma Scale (GCS) is used to determine the level of a conscious state. The lowest score is a three, and the highest is a fifteen. In the emergency room after the accident, Jessica was at a level four. She was a three while comatose, but she has been hovering around a level nine since she began waking up. Wiggling her toes when asked indicates that she understands what is being asked of her and can respond to it, meaning her score increases.

"The thing is, Ms. Lavine, she has not been able to show us the same response when we repeat the test. She hasn't wiggled her toes again."

"No, but she has smiled for and reached for her dance coach! She tried to lift her head for her riding instructor! She smiled at her cousin Hannah last night and was moving her mouth when her aunt and I were talking, as if she wanted to join in on the conversation! I see her in there! I know she is aware. I know she is in there."

The team shifts uncomfortably in their seats while the pediatrician tries to make me understand why those things aren't good enough. "But we haven't seen that, Ms. Lavine."

"It has happened."

I don't understand why they don't believe me or what I can do to prove to them that Jessica is more than alive. She is aware. She is in there, listening to us and understanding what we are saying. It's huge that she followed the doctor's command at all, but she has never been a monkey who will dance when asked. She is going to do her own thing when she is damn good and ready. The responses she makes for the loved ones in her life hold more meaning for me than whether or not she will wiggle her toes or blink her eyes for people she doesn't know and who obviously don't even believe in her.

There has to be something I can tell them to win them over. To make them believe in my girl.

It hits me. "Nicole!"

Nicole jumps a bit in her seat and looks at me, confused.

I plead with her. "You know. You've seen it. You know what I'm talking about."

As Jessica's physical therapist, Nicole has been working with my daughter for the two weeks we have been in The Pit of Despair. Jessica responds to her very well. Her spirit lightens when Nicole walks into the room. When Nicole is working with her arms or legs and Jessica begins to grimace, Nicole simply teases her about her "stink face," and Jessica calms down.

The other day, the surgery to have Jessica's G-tube placed conflicted with Nicole's regularly scheduled time. It didn't stop her from popping in to see Jessica before the surgery. She sat on the bed, chatting with Jessica before the transfer team came to wheel her down to the surgical floor. When the nurse came in and told us it was time to go, Jessica's face immediately scrunched up in her stink face. She was obviously upset. If she were capable of crying at that point, I'm sure she would have done so.

As much as my heart broke to see her scared and upset, *on some level* she understood the plan for the day. She was scared and expressed it. Once back from surgery, she was moaning more and trying to cry. She didn't quite get the gumption up to push her tears all the way out, but she gave a good effort.

I remind Nicole of all of this, and she nods. "She definitely had a reaction. I'd have to agree that she understood what was going on and wasn't happy about it."

I release the breath I've been holding and look expectantly at the doctors again.

"Well, that's good information to have," the pediatric doctor states. The neurosurgeon nods in agreement.

I simply stare, disappointed in their lack of faith. I'm dangerously close to turning over the table and storming out of the room. "Great. Now what?"

I slump back in my chair and listen to them discuss the dry details of Jessica's case: Visitor restrictions are lifted. She's out of the "acute" waking stage. We need to work on regulating her circadian rhythms and creating a more normal sleep schedule. The staples in her head have been removed. The swelling and discoloration of her right eye are 99 percent gone, and her right eye has begun responding to light when the doctors examine her.

She is still on one antibiotic for an infection. She is on a beta blocker to help with her "storming," an antacid to help with stomach acids, probiotics and Difulcan for a severe case of thrush, and potassium and sodium to regulate her electrolytes.

While it sounds like a lot, it is certainly less than the seventeen IVs she was on at the beginning of this ordeal. If any one of the meds she is taking now were stopped, it wouldn't pose an immediate threat to her life. She is breathing on her own and no longer needs respiratory therapy. The only monitoring they are doing now measures her blood pressure, heart rate, oxygen saturation, and respiratory rate.

The pediatrician glances around the table at his colleagues and clears his throat. "Is this all to say that Jessica is ready to be discharged?"

Silence hangs in the room as I stare at him. I close my eyes and start to count the seconds, having lost the capability of speech in this unbelievable moment.

One Mississippi. Two Mississippi.

How can she be ready? Three Mississippi.

She's not better. Four Mississippi.

How will we care for her? Five Mississippi.

Questions and thoughts crowd into my brain. When I make it

to ten Mississippi, I open my eyes to find most of the room looking at me expectantly. I open my mouth to speak, but all that comes out is a string of breathless sounds. Time starts again, and everyone begins talking at once.

CHAPTER FOURTEEN

One of My Kind

This cold metal bench is a far cry from the safety of my warm bed, where I can retreat under the covers and hide from the world, but I suppose it'll have to do for now. I lean back and look up at the blue, cloudless sky, trying to shake off the last moments of the Family Meeting from which I've escaped.

The doctors' words continue on an endless loop in my mind, and I stretch my arms upward while inhaling deeply. I then slowly bring my arms down and bend forward, forcing myself to push the air out of my lungs. Forcing myself to breathe.

"C'mon, let it go," I mumble to myself as I continue to bend forward, finally bringing my elbows to rest on my knees and cradling my head in my hands.

While lost in the task of drawing each breath, time slipped away. I'm not sure how long I've been sitting here before I realize my phone is ringing. I check the caller ID. It's Kathy.

"Hey."

"Hey, darlin'. How are you doing?" Kathy lives in Texas by way of Oklahoma by way of New York by way of Philadelphia. Her accent is tinged with a raw, rough edge that matches her personality, but underneath that edge is a softness that comes through in times like these. I take instant comfort in the familiarity of her voice, and all I can do is sigh in response.

I hear the unmistakable exhale of cigarette smoke on her end, and I squeeze my eyes shut and beg the world to stop spinning. Any comfort I thought I'd found on this metal bench has evaporated.

"I'm…I…" My breath bursts forth as I struggle to answer her question. *How am I doing?*

"I know, honey. I know."

The tears finally come. These are the tears I have been holding onto since I slid into the dirt. Even over a phone line, separated by a thousand miles, I feel safe in the intimacy and strength of the friendship we share. Though we've not had much "real-life" interaction, twelve years of daily communication in online chat rooms, emails, and the many social networking sites that have come and gone have left me feeling closer to Kathy than many people I see in "real life".

She was in my wedding, and I saved her from a dismal Valentine's weekend one year, when we both got tattooed. And here and now, as I struggle to put *how I'm doing* into words, I am sure she understands everything behind my sobs.

She exhales again. "Do you need me to come?"

The silence goes on too long, and I realize she can't see my head, which is bobbing up and down in response to her question. I push a simple "yes" into the phone with all my might.

"Okay." I hear her fingers flying over the keyboard. "Damn. Okay, I can probably only come for the night. There's no flight on Friday after work, and the flight on Saturday would get in at five. I would have to leave at nine on Sunday, because there's no later flight, and I have to work on Monday."

The reality of what she is saying shakes me from my meltdown, and I find my voice. "But that's only…"

"About twelve hours together after traveling to and from the airports. I know, but you need me."

"Are you sure?" I ask weakly, not wanting to have her fly halfway across the country to give me a twelve-hour hug but really wanting her to fly halfway across the country.

"Of course I'm sure. It's booked. Just get through the next week, and I'll be there."

"Okay." My breathing begins to stabilize.

"Okay." She takes a deep breath. "So, how are you doing?"

At this, I laugh and laugh. "Oh, honey. I can't wait to see you."

"Me, too."

The next week flies by in a blur of monitors, medications, and working to learn the ins and outs of Jessica's care and recovery. The Family Meeting the previous week ended with the doctors declaring Jessica ready to be discharged home, but Jesse and I argued that it's not possible when she's not better. We are untrained and unprepared to care for her at home. Not to mention the fact that we don't have the type of equipment necessary for her care and have no idea how to get it, since they told us it is not covered by our insurance. By the end of the meeting, I felt faint.

Nicole helpfully suggested that we see about getting transferred back to UCD for rehab evaluation and parental training. Now we're waiting to hear if UCD has a bed for Jessica and if they will accept the transfer.

By the time Kat arrives, I'm a frazzled mess, ready to download my thoughts and emotions directly into her brain. I am reluctant to leave the hospital, so Jesse takes Jocelyn and runs out to the airport. When they get back, I hug Kat tightly. She barely has a moment to sit with Jessica before Jocelyn is spinning, spinning, spinning through the room and ready to go back into the hall, get back in the car, and go go go.

So we go.

Once we're buckled in and heading to the house, I roll down the window and breathe in the fresh air.

"How are you doing?" Kat picks up the conversation right where we left it on the phone a few days prior.

"Oh, I am so glad you're here. You are one of the few people who can hold me up as I leave my heart lying in that hospital bed. I never would have left the hospital on my own, and, really, if I hadn't, I was either going to kill someone, or they were going to have to escort me out."

"What? I thought you were so happy with their care."

"Oh, no no no. I'm sorry." I can barely control the contempt in my voice as I explain the situation to Kathy. "That wasn't UC Davis."

Kathy rips the visitor sticker off her shirt and looks at it for the first time. "Oh."

"Yeah."

"When did this happen?"

"Two weeks ago. UC Davis determined Jessica to be stable enough to be transferred from the PICU onto the regular pediatric floor—"

"That's good, right? Does that mean she's progressing?"

I sigh, close my eyes briefly, and shake my head. "I don't really know anymore. In theory, I guess she is. The point is since she was stable enough to transfer to the regular pediatric floor, she was stable enough not to require the care of UC Davis Children's Hospital. So they transferred us to our HMO's facility."

"And that's . . . ?"

"The Pit of Despair, honestly."

"Oh, honey!" Kathy laughs the laugh saved for these dark situations. With her, it feels right, and I reach over and turn up the radio. Tears stream down our faces as we sing at the top of our lungs about how faith has been broken and tears must be cried.

Singing, laughing and crying with someone who sometimes understands me better than I understand myself allows me the first glimpse of the light at the end of the tunnel in this journey. Between her sweet laughter and singing through our tears, I can feel the healing light drift out into The Universe and trail behind us as we head for home.

When we reach the house, I pull into the driveway, put the car in park, and leave it running. We sit in the car for a minute, looking at the place I haven't stepped foot in for a month.

"It's been a month today," I murmur.

"I know, baby."

"There has to be a million dollar idea in here somewhere." I sigh.

"What do you mean?"

"This house. When we bought it, we weren't entirely sure it was big enough, yet for the past month I've been living in fifty square feet in the hospital. There has to be some sort of how-to marketing idea there, don't ya think?"

"Mmmm." She simply stares along with me.

"Out? Home? Go?" Jocelyn shakes us from our thoughts, and I turn off the car and set about unbuckling her and heading into the house.

"What's that?" Kathy points to the lock box hanging on the front door, as I unlock the doorknob with my house key.

"Lock box. My friend Cyndi quickly assembled Jessica's Posse, as she's calling it. There's a schedule out there somewhere listing when our trash needs to be carried to the curb, whose turn it is to bring Jesse and Jocelyn food, who will water our lawn and feed the animals, blah blah blah. They installed the lock box to avoid having to make twenty copies of the key."

"Wow. That's just..."

"Right?"

"Yeah."

We drop our purses on the table, and Jocelyn runs off to the toy room in search of her latest treasure. I look around for a minute, taking in the space and trying not to get lost. Our dog, Sugar, wags her butt at me, and I soak in the attention. I then set off to find the cats while Kathy makes herself busy in the kitchen.

Hours later, I ease myself out of my bed, in which Jocelyn has fallen asleep. I find Kathy in the living room. A pile of scrapbooks surround her, and she has a beer in her hand.

"You're brilliant," I tell her, opening the fridge to find a drink of my own. I splash some Seagram's and Sprite into a glass, take a long draw, and then refill it before joining my friend on the couch.

"That was a productive few hours," she states simply.

"Yeah, not exactly what I thought I'd be doing when I came home. Why did I jump into my least favorite jobs?"

"Which ones were those?" She cocks her head at me.

"The cat boxes, the guinea pig cage, the sweeping and mopping. I usually do laundry or dishes first. Thanks for cleaning out the fridge."

"Of course. All I really did was move a lot of stuff to the freezer. They are taking really good care of you guys. You have to see this." She pulls out a binder she has stashed between her leg and the couch. While she continues to browse through scrapbooks of our life before, I scan the *Lavine Family Care* binder. I read notes the members of "Jessica's Posse" have written to communicate what's been done and what might need to be done. Along with messages stating, "This week is recycling week." and "Can someone pick up bedding for the guinea pig cage?" are notes of love and prayers for our family.

As I lose the battle against the tears that are welling up, Kathy reaches out and takes my hand in hers. I am struck by the importance of having someone here with whom I feel completely safe. I don't need to worry about holding myself together anymore. I finally break a little, aware that I'm in good hands.

Morning comes far too quickly. I take an honest-to-goodness real shower, hustle to get Jocelyn ready, and repack my hospital bag with clean clothes, snacks, and the stack of mail from the kitchen counter.

Before we leave for the airport, I check my email and Facebook. An entry from Kathy is one of the first things in my feed.

If any of Jolene's local crew happen to see this, I want to thank you. Thank you for visiting Jessica, for keeping in touch with Jolene and Jesse, for taking care of the dog and the cats and the guinea pigs and the snake and for leaving notes of what you'd done. Thank you for vacuuming and doing dishes and making sure the doors are locked. Thank you for loving my friend as much as I do. The things you're doing are making it so much easier for Jolene to focus her energy and attention on Jessica and her treatment and make clear-headed decisions.

And to those of you in the far-away, long-distance-friend gang like me, I don't think you can possibly overestimate how much Jolene needs to keep hearing from people, talking to people, having things to do. Her world has necessarily become very small, and for hours every day it's just Jolene and Jessica in a hospital room with Wi-Fi and an iPhone. Keep in touch.

I shut down the computer and gather my things, and we head out the door. Door locked, I drop my bags and pull Kathy into a fierce hug. "Thank you," I whisper.

"I love you," she whispers back.

"Obviously."

CHAPTER FIFTEEN

Sepia-Toned Loving

Feeling a bit more rested and somewhat refreshed, I return to the hospital and am greeted by Jesse with great news.

"We're going back to UC Davis."

"When?" I set Jocelyn down on the chair-bed, kiss Jesse quickly, and then slide over to Jessica's bed. She turns her head a fraction of an inch toward me, and the corners of her mouth twitch. "Hi, baby! Yes, I'm here. I'm sorry I was gone. I missed you."

She blinks slowly a few times, and I stroke her hair and kiss her face, forgetting the news Jesse shared with me.

"I'll take Jocelyn to the cafeteria," he says. "I can talk to you when I come back."

"Okay, honey. Thanks." Grabbing a bottle of lotion from the drawer of the nightstand, I begin my routine of massaging Jessica's arms, legs, hands, and feet while chatting to her about the date, where we are, how she is doing, and how very much I love her.

"We're going to take another ambulance ride to UC Davis, and we'll go home after that. What do you think? Will it be better to be home?"

She blinks again, and I look in her eyes. Seeing her in there. HER. My sweet little Soul. She's floating, barely out of reach. To grab the invisible cord and pull her to me, I sit, massaging, chatting, meditating, praying, corralling energy, and simply willing her to heal.

When her eyes grow heavy, I encourage her to sleep. I feel that's what she's really doing, rather than being in a drug-induced coma, sedated, or crashed out on pain meds.

Jesse returns with Jocelyn, and we work to entertain her quietly on the small window seat in the far corner of the room while Jesse tells me the plan for our move.

He repeats what he's been told by the doctors. "As soon as they have a bed open up, we'll be on our way."

"And how long will we be there?"

"They made it sound like only a few days, while they teach us about her care and evaluate her for rehab."

Jocelyn plays with some blocks, and I squeeze Jesse's hand. "When will my girl come back to me?"

He squeezes my hand in reply. "I don't know. I wish I did."

"She's already come so far. She was so close to death. She still has so far to go."

"But she is coming back. She is waking up more and more every day. The storming really sucks, but I feel like every time she storms, something else clicks."

"You noticed that too?" I ask as I meet his eyes and we share a small smile. "It's weird. Things like that are so scary, but what they mean for her recovery is very encouraging."

"Right. While you were gone, the doctor said Jess is becoming more susceptible to stimuli, which sucks, but that also means she is becoming more aware! It's such a double-edged sword."

Jessica sleeps on peacefully, and I'm hypnotized by the sight. "She seems to be making some big and important steps. I am proud of her and excited about each new change, but damn... my impatience."

"A thing of legends, darling." He is teasing me gently. As Jocelyn climbs up into his lap with a book, I playfully swat his arm.

"I can't help it. I can't wait to have her up and walking, talking, dancing, and giggling again." I pause to rub my eyes. "I can't wait for this nightmare to be over. Time is moving much quicker now than it did in the beginning, but we're returning to UCD. How many days are left before I'm able to sleep in my own bed agai on my own couch? Have dinner together?"

Jesse divides his attention between turning pages for Jocelyn and rubbing my shoulder.

"I don't regret the time I spend here with her, but I miss having our family together. I'm scared for our future and how this will truly affect all of us. I'm so grateful we have a strong family unit and seem to be flying through this together, but we're so fractured right now. I'm saddened by the fact that I don't know when it will end."

He moves closer to me, and I reach out to take Jocelyn from him. She struggles to keep her legs in Jesse's lap. We sit like this, sharing our littlest child, while our big girl heals.

"Even though it's scary to think about going home," he tells me, "I'm eager to be there. If there is nothing to be done for her medically, I'd rather have her in an environment that is familiar to her."

"Yeah." His logic usually wins over my emotions. "Having us all together again and being surrounded by her things, the animals, everything she knows—"

"That can only impact her recovery in a positive manner."

"Just have to hope it doesn't take too long. It's draining and tiring, but I have to have faith in the beauty of The Universe and the fact that miracles happen every day. She's already proven that."

"Yeah, we have a lot of work cut out for us."

"We do."

"We can do it. Together."

"Absolutely." I lay my head on his shoulder. "Together, there isn't anything we *can't* do."

CHAPTER SIXTEEN

Every Little Thing They Do

"Good evening, Ms. Lavine." Jessica and I are getting settled into our room at UCD when a tall, brown-haired doctor enters the room, holding his hand out to me. "I'm Dr. Gerritz, a resident on the PM&R service."

"PM&R?" I'd heard the term at The Pit, but it never sank in enough for me to understand. If they'll be using it here at UCD, as well, I guess I better start our stay by asking the right questions and keeping the control we've managed to gain over Jessica's care.

"Physical Medicine and Rehabilitation. We're the department that will oversee Jessica's care. We will be evaluating her for rehab and determining her goals over the next couple of weeks."

"Weeks? We were told we would only be here for a few days."

Dr. Gerritz reviews his notes, and I take the opportunity to grab my notepad and a pen so I can jot a few notes of my own. On the nights Jesse isn't able to make it to the hospital, we chat on the phone before bed. Taking notes about the conversations in the hospital makes it easier to give him a daily update.

"Well, I'm not sure what you were told, but rehabilitation stays are usually more than just a few days. There's not much we can do in such a short amount of time."

"Okay. That's obviously fine. Our HMO hospital told us that we would be coming here for parent training and rehab evaluation. They made it sound like it would be only a few days before we would go home."

"I'm not sure why they told you that. We don't really have a parent training class here. Part of Jessica's rehabilitation will involve training your family on exercises for her at home; however, it's not any kind of formal class."

"Huh. Well, that's weird. Or I guess it makes sense given how things progressed there. Anyway... so what is the plan for Jessica then?"

Dr. Gerritz drops his notes into the pocket of his lab coat and begins to examine Jessica. I'm shocked by the aggressive way he handles her body. Before I can ask him to be more gentle, I'm stopped by the look on Jessica's face.

She appears to have been caught by surprise, as well, but she has a look of *interest* on her face. Her eyes are wide, and she is more aware than I've seen her since she began waking up weeks ago.

"Because you arrived here so late, she won't get her evaluations until tomorrow. A physical therapist, occupational therapist, and speech therapist will be in to evaluate her. Each will write a treatment plan and determine some goals for her." He continues to move her arms and legs and then tests her reflexes. He performs a quick eye exam, shining a light in Jessica's eyes and asking her to follow his finger. From where I'm sitting, I can't tell if what her eyes are doing is a good thing or a bad thing.

Dr. Gerritz retrieves his notes and begins writing quickly. "In addition to the therapists, Dr. Manhart, the PM&R attending, will stop in tomorrow. He will probably discuss the possibility of starting Jessica on a couple of new medications."

"What type of medications?"

"There are neurostimulants we can prescribe that will help her be a little more alert, as well as antispasticity medication to improve her muscle tone."

"We've been holding off on any kind of medication. I want Jessica to have the chance to recover as much as she can on her own."

"I understand. The point of the medications will be to avoid something called contractures. Should Jessica's muscle tone continue to be as tight as it is now, it will cause shortening of the muscles and stiffening of the joints, which will be very difficult to correct. While the medications are aggressive, realistically, it may be the best avenue for her."

I'm a little alarmed at the return of the "realistic" picture being painted for us. "Do I have time to discuss this with my husband before making a decision?"

"Absolutely. Jessica's situation is not dire right now. We can discuss it when Dr. Manhart is here in the morning."

"I just... is her progress slow right now? We'd like to avoid anything unnecessary." I move close to the side of Jessica's bed, take her hand, and rub her forehead gently.

"I understand. Again, it isn't a decision that needs to be made tonight, but it is something we should discuss to give Jessica every chance to recover as much as she possibly can. Unless she makes a dramatic turn for the better, it wouldn't be realistic to assume your family is prepared for the amount of time and therapy her body will require without the medication. It would border on unrealistic for any therapy team."

Despite what feels like the brutal honesty of his words, the tone in Dr. Gerritz' voice begins to soften the hard edges of my attitude. I've spent the past three and a half weeks battling doctors, trying to make them believe in Jessica's ability to recover. I haven't yet had the opportunity to acclimate myself to the attitude of possibility that Dr. Gerritz is presenting. I swallow hard and hold out my hand to him again. "Thank you, Doctor. I'll talk to my husband tonight and look forward to meeting Dr. Manhart in the morning. It was nice to meet you."

"You too." He shakes my hand and turns to Jessica. "Good night, Jessica. Get some rest so you'll be ready to work in the morning."

I watch him leave and then pull up Jessica's covers and arrange her pillows a bit, trying to make sure she's as comfortable as possible for the night. I pull out the all-too-familiar chair-bed. Instead of fooling myself into thinking I will be able to fall asleep anytime soon, I pick up my phone and text Kari for advice.

We got to UCD a little bit ago. Do you know Dr. Gerritz and Dr. Manhart?

I don't recognize Dr. Gerritz, but Dr. Manhart is one of the best, if not the best, physiatrists in our area.

Oh, okay. We'll be meeting him in the morning. Dr. Gerritz was here tonight and broached the subject of starting Jessica on some medications? What do you think?

I don't know who Gerritz is; is he an attending? Dr. Manhart is the best. I would trust whatever he says. He's going to do all he can to bring Jessica back to us. What room are you in? We'll be by to visit tomorrow afternoon.

Good. It'll be good to see you. I'd like to discuss what they say in the morning.

Of course, honey. Han and I will see you then. Love you. XO

Love you. XOXOXOXOXO

CHAPTER SEVENTEEN

A Little Hope in a Little Girl

I wake up early enough for a quick shower before getting Jessica cleaned up and changed. Dr. Gerritz never told me what time he and Dr. Manhart or the therapists would arrive. I assume it will be no earlier than 8:00 or 9:00, but it won't hurt for us to be up and ready anyway.

"Here they are." A blonde nurse comes through the door, followed by Jesse, who bears the gift of a Starbucks breakfast. While he hugs me, the new nurse writes on the nursing board at the end of Jessica's bed.

Jesse hands me my usual chai latte and kisses me before turning to say hello to his other girl.

The nurse says hello to her, too. "Good morning, Jessica. My name is Laurie, and I'll be your nurse today." She glances at me while plugging in the cart that holds the blood pressure cuff and oxygen monitor. "How was her night, Ms. Lavine?"

"Jolene, please. It seemed to be okay." I scan the nursing board, which is different from the ones they used in the PICU. This one has a note at the top: *This board will be used by your nurse. Together you will write down goals for you and your child.* In addition to the goals section, there is a spot for the primary and shift nurses to write their names. I note that Laurie has added her name as both the primary and the shift nurse.

"What is the difference between a primary nurse and a shift nurse?"

"I'll be Jessica's primary nurse, which means any time she comes here, I'll be assigned to her. It helps provide continuity of care."

"Oh, okay. So, the shift nurse is whoever is on for the day?"

"Yes. We have twelve-hour shifts, seven to seven. I'll be here until this evening." She puts the blood pressure cuff around Jessica's arm and tells her softly, "Just a little squeeze, Princess." My heart melts.

Jesse smiles a little and shakes his head, indicating that he knows what I'm thinking: *I love her already!*

We hear a gentle knock on the door and Laurie reaches over to open it. A woman from the Child Life department sticks her head in. "I thought I recognized your name on the list."

"Ms. K! Come in!" I hop up to give our new visitor a quick hug. While we were in the PICU immediately after the accident, Ms. K provided Reiki services to Jessica. Reiki is a Japanese technique for stress reduction and relaxation that also promotes healing. I'm grateful UCD offers this service, as Reiki is a small part of our beliefs about energy work and the power of positive thinking for healing.

I relay the news to Jessica. "Honey, Ms. K, the Reiki lady, is here."

Ms. K leans over the side of Jessica's bed to greet her. "Jessica, we haven't actually had the pleasure of meeting. I'm Ms. K, and it is so good to meet you."

In that moment, I realize the people at UCD who might remember Jessica haven't seen her for three and a half weeks. They haven't seen her without all of the IVs, without her NG tube, without the staples in her head, or without all of the monitors. They haven't seen HER. More and more, I am looking forward to our new time here.

There's another knock at the door, and a young woman joins us at Jessica's bedside. She wears glasses, and her long brown hair is pulled into a ponytail. "Hi, I'm Trish, the physical therapist. This must be Jessica."

I nod at her while waving to Ms. K, who is quietly exiting the room. "I'll see you later," she whispers. I mouth a "Yes, please!" to her.

I turn to the bed to see Trish giving Jessica the same type of aggressive evaluation Dr. Gerritz performed the night before. Again,

Jessica doesn't seem disturbed by this, but she appears to be more interested in what this woman is doing to her. She follows Trish with her eyes the best she can.

"Has Jessica been in bed the entire time she's been in the hospital?"

"No. When we were at the other hospital, they put her in a cardiac chair a handful of times. I think they had her up to sixty degrees."

"Well, we'll see if we can't do a little better than that. Okay?" I step aside and sit on the edge of the chair. Trish drops the side of Jessica's bed and begins maneuvering Jessica's body gently. I glance at Jesse, who moves closer to me, putting his hand on my shoulder and squeezing.

Within seconds, Trish has rolled Jessica onto her right side. She pulls her legs closer to the side of the bed and squats down a bit; then, in one swift motion, she has Jessica sitting on the edge of the bed.

"Nnnnnnnggggghhhhhhhhhh!" Jessica lets out a long moan, and then her mouth hangs open in a wordless yell. I lurch forward, hands reaching, but check myself, not wanting to disturb the work Trish is doing. I'm breathing heavily, and tears roll down my face.

Trish smiles at me gently. "It's okay to touch her."

That's all it takes. In a second, I'm next to Jess, my arm around her, letting her lean into me while I cry into her broken head. "You're doing great, baby girl. You're doing just fine. Mommy and Daddy are here, and you are so strong."

We sit like this for a few minutes before Trish indicates we should lay her down. "She is very strong. We will be working on getting her up more and more." She takes a folded page from her scrub pocket and makes a few notes. "They want to take her down to the vascular lab now to check her for blood clots, so either I or someone else from PT will come for Jess this afternoon."

Our morning evolves.

The nurses transport Jessica to the vascular lab and then return her to her room, where another physical therapist, a kind gentleman named Jack, is adjusting a wheelchair. We learn it will be used to transport Jessica to and from her therapy sessions, which will take place in a pediatric gym rather than in her hospital room.

As soon as Jessica is settled into her new ride, Jesse takes her for a walk around the floor while Holly, the social worker, and I talk about Jessica's injury and our family history. She provides a little more information about our stay in rehab and the services and resources available to us.

When Jesse and Jessica return, they are followed through the door by Dr. Gerritz and a tall, dark-haired doctor sporting a goatee. I do a double take, because if he were wearing glasses, he would look just like Dr. Pretzlaff from the PICU.

"Good morning, Jessica. I'm Dr. Manhart." A chill runs down my spine as I remember the evening texts between Kari and me. This is the doctor with whom she would willingly entrust her niece's care. I'm speechless for the moment, holding my breath and waiting for him to finish his exam of our girl.

"So... medication?" He looks at Jesse and me, and I look at Jesse, panicked. So much has been going on that I haven't had a chance to tell him about the conversation Dr. Gerritz and I had the previous night.

"I... we're not sure," I reply. "I'm sorry. We haven't had the chance to discuss it yet."

"Well, I would highly recommend it. Jessica's tone is very tight and will only get worse from here. The AFOs and PT can only do so much for now. I would recommend giving her a couple of shots of Botox right into the muscle, which will help relax them a bit, and then put her on baclofen—"

"Botox? The face drug?"

"It's actually a nerve impulse blocker. It prevents the release of the chemical transmitters that are making her muscles so tight."

"How often would she have to get those shots?"

"They're usually good for three to six months. By that time, she may not need another shot. If she's up and around and responding positively to physical therapy, this may be a one-time thing."

I straighten up and step toward the bed, eyes fixed on this man's face. I have only known him for ten minutes, but I will give him the world if he can return mine to me. "You think she will recover?"

He leans on the rail of Jessica's bed, lifts her arm, and gives it a wiggle. The way he moves our girl doesn't seem to be an exam as much as him just messing around. "What do you think, Jessica?"

He shakes her legs a little and then pushes on her shoulder. I watch Jessica's face and would swear I can read her thoughts in the glimmer of her eye and the twitching in her mouth. It's the face she makes when her dad tells her she's grounded for the smallest infraction or when I tell her she can't bring a book to read in the car when we're going on a long drive. It's the look she gives us when she knows we're not serious, and she wants to say, "Stop teasing me!"

"Doctor?"

He smiles at me, shakes his head, and lifts his hands. "We can't predict anything with certainty, but we've seen some amazing things happen. What I want to do is give Jessica the best chance she has. I believe the medications we want to give her will help. She won't have to be on them forever. We will reevaluate as she progresses, but I think they are necessary now."

I barely look at Jesse before nodding and giving my consent. "Let's do it, then. Thank you, Dr. Manhart."

"You're welcome. Get ready to work hard, Jessica. Let's see what you can do."

As he and Dr. Gerritz leave the room, I move to the head of the bed and pull Jessica into a hug as much as I can and kiss her face all over. "You heard him, baby. I know you can recover; I know you can be well. I love you, baby girl."

We have only a moment like this before two more therapists enter the room. "It's a party in here," I whisper to Jesse as I look at our new guests expectantly.

"Is this Jessica?" Short brown hair and a green backpack slung over her shoulder, one of the women checks her notes before putting them into her scrub pocket.

I respond to her question. "This is she."

"Jessica, I'm Faye. I'm an occupational therapist, and I've heard so much about you."

"I'm Kristin. I'm a speech therapist. Jessica's schedule has been a bit busy this morning, so if you don't mind, Faye and I want to double up on our evaluation."

"No problem at all. Of course, whatever works."

"Has she been responding to any commands at all?" Faye asks as she sets down her backpack and lowers the side of the bed.

"Here and there." I sit on the edge of the chair-bed again so there will be enough room for both therapists to evaluate Jessica. "Her dad and I can tell she's aware, but it's that kind of thing, you know? Where it's really easy for us to tell. She's only responded to a couple of commands. She does react to people, though. She's reached for her dance coach and smiled for her cousin . . . those sorts of things."

Faye nods along while she and Kristin work together to sit Jessica up on the side of the bed again.

"Has she been holding her head up at all?" Kristin asks.

"Umm, not too much, I guess. She was only out of bed a few times at the other hospital and then this morning when the physical therapist did her evaluation. Was her name Trish?"

"Yep. We did talk to her."

"Yeah, and then Jack. He set up her wheelchair."

"Ah, Señor Jack." Faye smiles while studying Jessica's face. Jessica studies her right back for a minute. I watch the two of them and then glance at Jesse. He raises his eyebrows, and I smile. *Something big is happening here.*

Faye and Kristin lay Jessica down again and ask us a series of questions regarding whether or not Jessica has had any regular food.

How is her oral care? Has she made any sounds to communicate? Is she able to do anything on her own yet?

The familiar sense of defeat and hopelessness washes over me as I answer their questions, mostly in the negative. As wonderful as it has been for Jesse and me to feel that Jessica is aware and understands what is going on, the questions from the medical professionals paint the all-too-familiar *realistic* picture for us. It's impossible to ignore how much Jessica hasn't recovered.

Faye and Kristin finish the evaluation and make their exit when Laurie comes in to start Jessica on her new medications. She also does her midday assessment and starts the feeding pump that sends Pediasure through a tube directly into Jessica's stomach.

Jesse leaves for a half day of work at the office. When the pediatric floor lights dim for rest time for the patients, I stare out the window, making occasional notes on the notepad. I write down the names, the information we've been given, and questions that occur to me as I sit in silence.

As soon as rest time ends, another flurry of activity begins. Faye shows up, a short board tucked under her arm.

"Are you ready to roll, kid?"

Jessica seems interested.

"So, Mom, this is a slide board. It's used to help get her from the bed into the wheelchair."

"Okay." I move to the end of the bed to position myself for a better view. Faye drops the side rail and pulls the wheelchair over so it is parallel and flush with the bed. She then maneuvers Jessica in what is becoming a familiar way, rolling her onto her right side, putting her legs over the side of the bed, and then sitting her up. I make a mental note to practice this while we're still in the hospital and under the watchful eye of the professionals.

Faye places the board as a connector between the bed and the wheelchair, wedging it under Jessica's bum a little.

"You ready, girl?" She looks into Jessica's face and must see an indication of a positive answer. She puts her hands under Jessica's armpits, braces Jessica's feet between her legs, and slides Jessica's bum along the board until it is in the seat. Jessica is sitting a bit crooked, but she has safely made the transition. It takes less than a minute for Faye to straighten Jessica's body and legs and buckle her in. Just like that, we're heading off the pediatric floor.

"The pediatric gym is down one floor and on the opposite side of the hospital," Faye tells me as she pushes Jessica toward the elevators at the end of the hall, moving at a rapid pace. "Once you're comfortable getting Jessica out of bed, it would save transport time if you can take her straight to the gym. Then we can use the full session for work."

I nod, rushing to keep up.

"Her normal schedule will be half an hour of occupational therapy, half an hour of physical therapy, and half an hour of speech therapy in the morning and again in the afternoon. They'll start bringing a schedule to your room the day before. And here we are."

The only clue we are "here" are puzzle pieces and farm animals painted on the wall in the short hallway. I see a door on the left wall, a door at the end, and a narrow hallway to the right that leads to two other doors. Faye unlocks the door before us, using a key that hangs off her lanyard along with her hospital ID and something labeled *Vocera*.

She flips on the light, and we enter a long room filled with therapy aids. A large treatment table is positioned at one end near cabinets that store balls, games, and bins. They are labeled not by content but by which area they work on: "fine motor," "gross motor," "tactile," and more.

We spend the next hour and a half in this room. Faye transfers Jessica to the table, where she works on stretching her muscles and measuring her range of motion. Kristin arrives at the gym as soon as Faye's time is up. Faye helps transfer Jessica to the wheelchair.

Kristin works to get Jessica to move her mouth and visually track objects. She asks Jessica to close her eyes and stick out her tongue. My heart sinks, as it's unclear whether Jessica hears and understands Kristin but *can't* do what is asked of her... or if she simply doesn't understand. Thirty minutes of discouraging progress creep by before Jack enters the room, pushing a long table with straps on it.

"Hey, Jessica!" He greets her with a big smile. Jessica's eyes are still alert, and she blinks at him. I thank Kristin and then move the chair I've been sitting on to allow Jack enough space to maneuver Jessica next to the table.

"We are going to try to get Jessica a bit more vertical today."

"Oh?" I bite my lip, nervous about how this might be achieved.

"Yeah, give me a second." He focuses his full attention on Jessica, bracing her legs between his legs and placing his hands under her armpits. In one swift movement, he lifts her from her sitting position and pivots her so her bum is sitting on the table.

"Wow." The process is less involved than using the slide board Faye showed me earlier, but it also seems to require some finesse. Both methods will take practice, I'm sure.

"Yeah? Haven't seen that one, huh?" Jack's manner is light and jovial, and I smile at him.

"Not yet. So... do you prefer Jack or Señor Jack?"

He glances at me and chuckles. "Oh, ho ho. Who's your mom been talking to, Jessica?"

I grin at him while he carefully lays Jessica on the table and connects the wide straps that go across her hips and her calves, securing her to the table. Jack turns a crank, and the table begins to move from a horizontal position to vertical. He continues to operate the crank until Jessica is "standing" at about a forty-five degree angle.

"The goal will be to eventually get her to ninety degrees," Jack says. "For now, we'll start slow. How is that, Jessica? Feel pretty good?"

She doesn't respond, of course, and I trust Jack's expertise to know whether she is capable of sustaining this position much longer.

"To help build the strength in your legs further, we can do squats, too." He helps Jessica bend her knees, which makes her slide down the table a bit. When he pushes her knees against the table, she is again standing straight up. He performs the maneuver a few more times, and memories of Melissa's ballet class are once again in my head. Tears fill my eyes.

"It's like a plié, sweetheart." I swear I see her eyes flicker in recognition. "Like you would do in Ms. Melissa's ballet class. Do you remember how to plié?"

Jack helps her plié again, though he seems a bit confused by the reference. "Well, sure, whatever works," he says. "It's all French to me."

I can't contain my laughter at his offhand comment. "Exactly!"

He shakes his head and gives me a quizzical look. I wave him away, saying, "Just a dance thing."

I lose myself in the memories of girls in black leotards and pink tights lined up at the barre, moving in unison as Ms. Melissa calls out the French terms for the moves they know by heart.

As our week progresses, we develop a fluidity in our schedule that carries us from one hour to the next. I get Jessica up each morning and make sure she's cleaned up, changed, and comfortable. I wash her face and brush her teeth before Jesse arrives with Starbucks for breakfast. The nurses do their assessments, and Dr. Manhart or the other PM&R physician, Dr. Davidson, round on Jessica. They speak softly about the encouraging signs they've seen since the one-time injection of Botox and the introduction of the neurostimulants and antispasticity medications Jessica is receiving routinely now.

Jesse joins me for the morning sessions, the two of us soaking in the way the therapists move Jessica and talk to her. We're learning the tricks they use to help her regain function of her body and her mind. Every day they introduce a new activity, and every day we see something different in her. We watch, support, learn, and hope it will all unlock the door and allow her to walk through.

The plan remains nebulous, as they seem to evaluate something different with our girl every single day. By the end of the first week, Jessica has responded enough to encourage a second week of rehab. Three hours of therapy, Monday through Saturday. If they can get anything out of her right now, they will.

As eager as I am to be home, I'm happy to continue sleeping on the chair-bed and enduring the flat pillows and scratchy blankets for two or three more weeks if it means she is waking up more and responding well to treatment. It will be worth it if it allows these magical people to bring my baby back to me sooner rather than later.

CHAPTER EIGHTEEN

Nothing Less Will Save the Day

June 10, 2010 – Six Weeks Post-Accident

It's Thursday. I thought this might be the first week I wouldn't be painfully aware, to the hour, that another week has gone by. I'm obviously wrong, as I'm frozen in my chair with tears leaking from the corners of my eyes. I alternate between staring at Jessica and glancing at the clock. Unable to move. Unable to do what needs to be done.

Jesse enters with our usual breakfast, and I start sobbing. He quickly sets everything down and leans over me, pushing my hair from my face. "Honey? What is it? Is Jess okay?" He turns to check on her and then turns to me.

"She's fine," I choke out. Coughing, I force myself to sit up, and Jesse brings me a box of tissues from the counter. "I don't know what's wrong with me. I can't move." I blow my nose and lie down again, burying my face in the pillow.

I hear Jesse moving about the room, murmuring to Jessica, followed by the sound of papers being shuffled.

"Her therapy is at 10:00 this morning?"

"I don't know." My voice is muffled as I wail into the pillow. I never even checked the schedule when it was dropped off last night.

"Well, go ahead and relax. I'll start getting her ready." And he does. As I let the tears flow, pausing ever so briefly to wipe my running nose, Jesse gets Jessica dressed, changed, and comfortable. He washes her face and brushes her teeth and talks things over with the nurse when she arrives for the morning assessment.

Together, they move Jessica to the wheelchair and prepare for her busy schedule while I sniffle away on the chair-bed.

"Do you want to go?" Jesse asks me gently as the time to leave for therapy grows closer.

"I can't." I finally emerge from the pillow to look at him.

"What is it?" He squeezes my hands gently.

"It's all of it. I'm on my fucking period. It's been six weeks today. I am so tired and frightened of the worst, and I need something to shift."

Jesse reasons with me. "She's doing more in each therapy session. She has more control over her responses and her body. The neurostims are working. You know she's more aware. Her eyes are brighter, and she's more aware of her surroundings."

"She's also more agitated and scared. I have to reorient her so often," I argue. I'm determined to find a valid reason for my breakdown.

"That means she's waking up more," he counters. "Her body is looser; it's easier for the therapists to stretch her."

"But they said her right calf and ankle are stuck and can't be fixed. What if she never dances again?"

He sighs, sits on the edge of my chair-bed, and asks gently, "If she recovers to a point that a contracture is the only thing wrong with her, would that be so bad?"

I look at him, trying to process that possibility.

He takes advantage of my lack of argument and continues. "What I see is her focusing more on everything. Even when she is more agitated, scared, and crying, I believe it's simply a sign of her frustration at her limitations. She is healing, and we need to help her keep fighting."

I sigh and concentrate on folding the tissues in my hand.

He adds more examples to support his viewpoint. "What about what she has done for other people? When Mallory visited and she smiled at her? Or smiling for Hannah? Reaching for Melissa? These aren't small things."

I scoff and look at him hard. "Really? Smiles? It's easy for you. You get to escape to work! You have Jocelyn to take care of and interact with! How did *my* day…no, my *life*…How did my life become nothing more than sitting in this hospital room, getting excited over the fact that our precious, vibrant, active, healthy, brilliant, funny, sweet, compassionate, sassy, smack-talking, moody ten-year-old *smiled*? People with infants experience more excitement." I slump deeper into the chair-bed, and Jesse reaches for my hand. I stare at him.

He drops his hand and checks the clock. "Well…"

"Yeah. Welcome to my world. Not knowing what to say. Not knowing what to do. Sure, she smiles, but the rest of my time is spent fighting to keep her comfortable while she is…what? Storming? Moody? Scared? Angry? I don't know! Her heart rate shoots up, and nothing I try works. I read to her, play music, put on a movie, talk to her, show her pictures of family and friends until, finally, I just pretend to ignore her."

"Pretend to ignore her?" He's obviously confused.

"I organize our growing pile of bills and all of the papers with all of the notes about her therapies, her medications, the appointments we need to make, and the next procedure she has to have. I 'ignore' her and keep watch on the monitor to make sure her heart rate is what? Normal? Low? Where it was before I couldn't comfort her? I don't know what I'm looking for anymore."

"You're looking for answers," he says softly.

I stare at him again, my mouth hanging open this time. I snap it shut and return to folding my tissues. "Yeah. I suppose you're right."

He stands up and kisses me on the head. "I gotta get her to therapy."

"I know." I grab his hand and hug him to me awkwardly. "Thank you for taking her."

"Of course."

They head out the door, and I set about cleaning up the room a bit. The nurse has brought in clean linens, so I remake Jessica's bed and return my bed to chair status. I go through the papers on the counter, stacking those I need to keep and throwing out wrappers and snacks that have gone bad. I push all of the dirty linens into the hamper.

I take the time to shower, letting the water wash away the salt from my tears, hoping to rejuvenate enough so Jesse can still make it to work.

I return to the pediatric floor in time to see Jesse pushing Jessica through the hall, a triumphant smile on his face when he sees me. I hold the door to the room open for him and ask, "How'd it go?"

He parks Jessica by the bed and takes me into his arms. "I wish you would have gone. You should have been there."

I wish something would shift.

"Trish got Jessica to lie on her stomach on the mat. With her leg up behind her, Trish was pushing on her toes, working to stretch the muscles. We were talking about the stretches to do at home when Trish stopped and looked at me."

"What happened?" I'm getting caught up in his excitement.

"Trish said, 'That's all her.' And when I looked at Jessica's leg, her foot was moving. She was fighting the stretch. Not big movements, but she was trying to move against the way Trish was pushing her foot. With her right leg!"

"What? Oh, my god!"

"Yeah, Trish says her legs are just tight and need to be stretched. She does *not* have any contractures!"

"Oh, my god," I repeat, moving to sit down again. Jesse stays with me, leaning on the wall next to the chair so he can keep hold of my hands.

"That's not all."

"What do you mean?"

I need something to happen.

"Faye and the speech therapist…you know I'm bad with names…"

"Kristin?"

"Right. They teamed up today. They were working on having her stick out her tongue and trying to get her to close her eyes while Faye counted to three. At first, she closed her eyes, and we couldn't tell if she was blinking or if she was trying to close her eyes the way they asked."

"Okay."

"Faye asked her to do it again, and Jessica closed her eyes again! She never kept them closed until Faye counted to three, but she kept trying. She closed them longer and longer each time."

I look at Jessica now, who seems worn out and tired, but she is definitely watching Jesse and me as we chat.

"Finally…"

"There's more?"

I need something to shift.

"Yes. Kristin asked Jessica to stick out her tongue, and Jessica tried!"

My eyes are filling with tears again, and I am speechless. I look from Jessica to Jesse, shaking my head slowly.

He squeezes my hands tight. "Hearing. Understanding. Responding! *She is healing.*"

"Today was the day," I whisper as the tears fall.

"What do you mean?"

"I wanted something to shift today. I wanted a bigger slice, a bigger piece, a bigger spark of hope to help carry us through."

"Well, you got it. I wish you had been there."

"Me too."

"They also gave us some news."

"What news?"

"Next Friday is our tentative discharge date."

"What? Why now? She's beginning to respond!"

"We only have so many rehab days available to us through our insurance. They're planning to get as much out of them as they can. Going home will give her a chance to advance more and will optimize her progress when she resumes rehab here. Also, they'd like her head put back together before they do more with her."

"That makes sense. Oh, my goodness. Next Friday, huh?"

"Probably. Are you ready?"

"More ready now than I was when they tried to shove us out of the Pit of Despair. These people have made us ready."

"I agree. Let's go home."

"Let's go home," I echo, standing up to hug him tight.

CHAPTER NINETEEN

That's How the Light Gets In

June 17, 2010

"Honey, we need to go." Jesse is holding the door to Jessica's room open, but I'm cemented to the floor at the side of her bed, helping Laurie finish getting Jessica more comfortable. This is code for changing Jessica's position in the bed, which has to happen every two hours. It involves putting on or removing her AFOs and managing her personal hygiene, such as bathing, toileting, and brushing her teeth.

"It's okay. I'll stay with her until I get called into another room." Laurie has switched to attempting to make *me* more comfortable. We have been in the hospital so long now that dozens of nurses have worked with Jessica, but Laurie is her primary nurse. It has added to the sense of familiarity, and I've enjoyed getting to know Laurie over the past few weeks. She also seems to have a pretty good read on me, though I'm sure she's been in her field long enough to recognize a stressed-out-mom-on-the-edge from a hundred yards away.

"I'll finish helping you here before I go. I don't mind." I ignore the look Laurie and Jesse exchange and continue pushing pillows under Jessica's legs, arms, and hips. It's an attempt to prevent the dreaded bedsores that can be so common in bedridden patients. Jessica has overcome enough setbacks in her recovery thus far, and I don't want her to have to deal with a nuisance like bedsores on top of everything else.

"Do you even know where we're going?" Jesse asks.

"Um, not incredibly sure. Holly told me the general area. I wrote it down."

"Where is it?"

I freeze and stare at him, recognizing his ploy now. Keeping me focused has always been one of Jesse's greatest strengths. He simply smiles back at me and looks at the pillow in my hand.

I turn back to the bed, place the last pillow under Jessica's shoulder, and lean in to whisper to her. I search her eyes for any sign of the recognition and understanding we're sure we've seen in the past few weeks. "Dad and I are going to a meeting. We will be back very soon. Laurie will be with you as long as she can. I love you."

I'm sure I see a glimmer of understanding. I kiss her gently before grabbing my purse and a pad of paper.

"Okay, let's go," I mumble to Jesse.

In response, he puts his arm around me and gently pushes me forward.

"So, where are we going?" he asks.

I quicken my steps to keep up with his brisk pace.

"The conference room on the fifth floor, east." I recite the information written on the pad of paper, which is a mess of notes scribbled on nearly every inch of space.

"Okay, and that's at the other end?" He sighs while punching the elevator button.

"Yes, the same end as the gym where they do her therapy."

The meeting is two floors down, at the opposite end of the hospital from the pediatric floor, which means we should have left as soon as Jesse urged me to leave, but I can't bring myself to feel guilty about it. I have a hard enough time leaving Jessica as it is.

"You should have started bugging me earlier." I blame him in a half-joking manner as we exit the elevator and rush through the cardiac ward, dodging nurses, carts, and linen bales throughout the corridor.

"You're right." He's taking it easy on me, aware of my fragile mood. "So, are they going to let us know when we're being released?"

As we round the last corner, I smile at him. "I hope so. I've been making a pest of myself with Jodie. I think if we figure out the transportation, we could be discharged tomorrow or Saturday."

"Oh, good. Let's hope so." Jesse opens the door to the conference room, and I stop short.

"Are we in the right spot?" I whisper to Jesse, overwhelmed at the sight of the conference room filled with a dozen people. Faye catches my eye and waves me in.

"Wow, much different, huh?" Jesse whispers back. We fumble through hellos and make our way around the large conference table to seats that have been reserved for us right in the middle.

I quickly take my seat and apologize. "I'm sorry we're late." Fishing a pen from my purse, I flip to a blank page in my notepad.

"That's okay." Dr. Gerritz speaks first. He's the doctor I first met with when we returned to UC Davis from The Pit of Despair. During the three weeks of dealing with doctors who didn't seem concerned about whether my daughter ever progressed beyond lying comatose in a hospital bed, Jesse and I had realized that we needed to gain control of Jessica's treatment.

When we returned to UC Davis, I had a chip on my shoulder the size of Rhode Island. I was exhausted but prepared to continue fighting for Jessica's recovery. That led me to approach my initial meeting with Dr. Gerritz with the same irritation and attempt to control the situation that I'd developed at The Pit. He set me straight and laid out the treatment process they had planned for Jessica. He readily shared his knowledge of her case, the procedures he recommended, why he recommended them, and *how they would help Jessica get better*. It was a welcome change that pulverized the chip on my shoulder within seconds.

This same no-nonsense attitude sets the tone for the day's meeting.

"Because there are so many of us, I think we should get underway. Let's introduce ourselves before we speak, and that should work fine."

As murmurs of assent float around the room, I allow myself to settle into my seat and listen.

"I'm Dr. Gerritz, resident physician of the Physical Medicine and Rehabilitation department. Today, we're discussing patient Jessica Lavine. She is a ten-year-old female who sustained a severe traumatic brain injury when she was kicked in the head by a horse at a horseback riding lesson. The impact resulted in significant fractures of her skull and brain damage in both hemispheres. Jessica has made great progress in her time here. She has been weaned off all of her sedatives and paralytics.

"Jessica suffers from aphasia and dysphasia. While we would like to know how her vision and hearing have been affected, we are holding off on those evaluations until Jessica is able to respond in a manner appropriate for the exams."

Dr. Gerritz pauses to take a breath and review Jessica's chart in front of him. I am in awe at the towering stack of paperwork on the table and grateful he can make sense of it all, helping us understand exactly what is happening with our child.

"Jessica has a severe case of thrush, for which she has completed meds, but she will need aggressive oral care over the next three to six months.

"She will also require surgery within the next three to six months to replace the missing bone flap.

"She is currently taking Ritalin, amantadine, baclofen, and Prilosec, but your own doctors may choose to adjust these medications. She received her final dose of fludrocortisone this week, as her salt-wasting is under control, and we are currently working to wean her off of the propranolol.

"In addition to Jessica's pediatrician and your PM&R Department, you will need to follow up with gastroenterology, pediatric ENT, audiology, and pediatric optometry. You will also need to contact your insurance provider to determine which durable medical equipment is covered.

"While we are concerned about the variations in Jessica's heart rate, her blood pressure is a better gauge of how she is handling the changes in her medications, and her blood pressure at this time is very good."

He shuffles through the medical records one last time and then looks at Jesse and me before he sums up his report.

"Jessica needs more time to recover in her own environment before returning to inpatient rehab. While you are eager to be in your own environment, and I agree it will help further this stage of Jessica's recovery, we need to look at the big picture. It is in Jessica's best interest to return to us for inpatient rehab. As I mentioned, follow up with your PM&R department. They'll probably set a telephone appointment first, within the next two weeks, but try to get into their clinic within the next four weeks.

"I think that's all I have. Do you have any questions for me?"

My head is spinning, and I look at Jesse to avoid voicing the only question that comes up for me: *When will this nightmare end?* At one point or another over the past seven weeks, I'm sure I've learned all of the information Dr. Gerritz just shared, but to hear it all laid out in such a succinct manner, with timelines and expectations, is both a blessing and a curse.

Jesse nods toward the notepad sitting in front of me, and I remember this is the first meeting for which I have prepared questions to have answered.

"Yes, the biggest question we have right now is regarding the bone flap surgery. Will that surgery be scheduled through our insurance company? They will be the ones to assess and determine when her bone flap should be replaced?"

"Yes. They will likely have Jessica come in for a CT scan so the prosthesis can be created. Once it's ready, they will schedule the surgery."

"Okay. Well, I think the other questions I have are for Jodie, so I'll wait."

Dr. Davidson, who is seated next to Dr. Gerritz, speaks next.

"Hi, guys, I'm Dr. Davidson, one of the attendings in the PM&R Department. I won't repeat everything Dr. Gerritz has reviewed. I want you to know that before you leave, we will make sure to draw up a complete list of appointments for you to request from your insurance company, as well as services to ask for, because they may not offer them."

"Wait, these services . . . will they be covered?" Jesse asks.

"They should be, but in our experience, they are not always offered by default. You will need to be more proactive with your insurance company. We won't have access to Jessica's records. We won't know when she's ready to come back for more therapy. You're going to have to make sure this happens."

I drop my pen, and Jesse and I stare at one another. The brief experience we had with our own hospital still stings like a fresh paper cut, and these doctors have just poured lemon juice on it.

We had hoped that the poor treatment we received from our own doctors could have been attributed to my high-strung mood, raw emotions, misplaced anger, and childish petulance. We naively believed things would be different after we returned to UCD for therapy evaluations and were discharged home. I am aghast that Dr. Davidson's experience with our insurance company confirms our fears that Jessica will not be properly treated through our own HMO.

"So what exactly do we need to do to get her the treatment she needs? The type of care you are giving her." Jesse has grabbed my hand and taken control.

Dr. Davidson's voice is soft and gentle. "Short of switching insurance companies, you will simply need to be on top of things. We will outline the list of appointments you need to ask for, as well as things to look for in Jessica, signs that will show that she may be ready to return to us for intensive rehab. We will help you as much as we can before you leave."

"Okay. What next, then? Do we know yet when we will be discharged?" I immediately regret the impatience in my voice, which shows how desperate I am for all of us to be in our own environment again.

Jodie pipes up. "Well, I don't want to go out of turn, but that's what I'm working on right now. I am trying to arrange for a bed and a suction machine to be delivered, but the most important piece is home health. Your insurance company doesn't have a home health nurse available, so we need to work with a contractor to set one up. That can take twenty-four to forty-eight hours, and—" She is interrupted by her phone ringing and holds up a finger, excusing herself to the hallway.

Since she showed up in one of Jessica's therapy sessions earlier this week, Jodie has impressed me with her efficiency. As the discharge planner, she found all of the balls that had been dropped when we were transferred back to UCD, and she has been helping me pick them up. She has been invaluable at guiding me through the discharge process.

"While she's on the phone, I'll go," Faye says. Thus begins the next hour of information overload. Faye explains the work we need to do to help Jessica regain as much use of her body as possible. She advises us about stretches designed to increase her range of motion, keep her wrists straight and her hands open, and prevent her hips from getting tight or her feet from dropping.

She emphasizes the point that in order to return to inpatient rehab, Jessica's responses must be consistent. She suggests we keep a log of response times when we ask Jessica to perform certain tasks, such as sticking out her tongue, raising her arms, or looking at specific objects. She advises us to talk Jessica through activities, engaging her in everything we are doing with her and the work we're having her do.

Faye continues. "Include her whenever you can, even if she's only in the kitchen with you while you are cooking. Have her sit at the table with you for meals. Play games with her, helping her reach the pieces and explaining each piece to her. Keeping her engaged is so important."

Toward the end of the overview, Faye lets us know that Jessica's sitting balance and head control are top priorities for returning to rehab.

At this point, everything feels like a top priority.

"I want to reiterate a lot of what Faye said." Trish, Jessica's physical therapist, is at bat now. She suggests we attempt to get a Hoyer Lift to help transfer Jessica from her bed to her wheelchair. Jesse and I have been doing a two-person lift, something that won't be sustainable once he is back to work full time. She also recommends working on a schedule for stretching Jessica's muscles. There is no time limit for Jessica to be in her wheelchair, but we are to watch for any signs of agitation, discomfort, or irritability. Trish advises us to keep an eye out for bedsores and skin breakdown, especially on Jessica's bony areas.

Kim, the speech therapist we haven't met yet, who is covering for Kristin today, nods along with her colleague's advice. "Routine, routine, routine," she hammers into us. "Tell her the date and what's happening. Encourage her to be active in games and family activities." She stresses the importance of the cognition side of things, helping Jessica understand all that is going on in the moment. She reminds us that helping Jessica with simple tasks will help her relearn cause and effect and how the world works.

Not only does speech therapy involve the cognitive piece of the puzzle but the oral aspect, as well. She echoes the urgency Dr. Gerritz expressed about her oral issues and advises that we get a tongue scraper, which will not only help clear the remnants of the thrush but will also stimulate Jessica's palate.

She tells us to purchase some sort of vibration tool to stimulate the exterior muscles of Jessica's face and to use Dum Dums suckers, Popsicle treats, and sour stimulation to promote saliva production and encourage Jessica's swallow reflex. She cautions us to keep an eye on Jessica's gag reflex and to be wary of her tonic bite, which can cause Jessica to involuntarily bite down on anything put in her mouth, creating a choking hazard.

As Kim is the last therapist to give her report, I consider putting my pen down and taking a breather. Before I have the chance, Holly, the social worker, hands me two pages stapled together.

"This is a list of agencies you can call to see about getting resources at your house. With all of the changes in state budgets and funding, things may have changed for a lot of them, but it's a place to start." She runs down the list of organizations and what each of them may be able to provide. I try to take notes, but my head is spinning again.

We receive more overwhelming information from the neuropsychologist when she talks about something called neuropsych testing, which will determine what functions and understanding Jessica has retained.

I wave her suggestion away. "I want her to have a chance to recover before testing her like that."

"Of course. I understand."

The last person to speak is the head nurse from the pediatric floor. She gives a short report about where things stand with Jessica's routine and medications.

I finally set my pen down and rub my eyes. I'm in awe of Jessica's medical team here. They have celebrated each of Jessica's successes to date and have shared their insights and guidance regarding what we can expect once we get home, as well as what we might hear from our insurance company.

They have suggested activities that we can do with Jessica in order to help push her forward in her recovery and have offered resources, tools, and websites to help accomplish that goal.

Dr. Gerritz breaks the silence. "I have to say that I have never seen a family fight so ferociously for the benefit of their child. Your passion will be your biggest asset as you move forward in this process. You will need that to be sure your daughter receives the services and treatment she deserves."

"Thank you." I am touched by his words and attempt to return them in kind. "Thank you for all you are doing. I don't understand why there is such a glaring difference in our experiences with you versus our experiences with our own insurance company." Overwhelmed, I take a drink of water and squeeze Jesse's hand.

Jesse clears his throat and picks up where I've left off. "It's obvious that you see Jessica's potential, and we appreciate how determined you are to pull it out of her. These successes you've mentioned . . . moving her finger, blinking her eyes, and moving her heel during a stretch . . . we never would have known to celebrate such things if we were still at our own hospital. That's not how they approached things."

As I look at each member of Jessica's team, I find a force to be reckoned with. A team of true professionals dedicated to the success of my child. I try to find my voice again, but it's no use. Voice cracking, I try to express my gratitude to them. "You believe in my girl and haven't counted her out. You don't see her as just another patient who happens to have a really bitchy and annoying mother . . ."

The room erupts in laughter, and Dr. Gerritz pushes a box of tissues toward me and reiterates his earlier sentiment. "You are advocating for your daughter."

"But you are, too. Thank you for believing in her." I pull a couple of tissues out of the box and wipe my eyes.

Jesse leans forward. "So, then, when do we get to leave?"

I lean forward eagerly, as well. My earlier doubts about our ability to care for our daughter have vanished. This team of experienced doctors and therapists has worked hard to train us and make sure we are comfortable with Jessica's daily routine. Moreover, they truly believe we will be able to do all that needs to be done in a setting that we all hope will push her closer to recovery.

Let's blow this Popsicle stand.

Jodie has been in and out of the meeting with phone calls. She enters the room and drops into her seat but avoids making eye contact with me. "We will have a bed delivered tomorrow, and I will continue to work on getting a suction machine and any other loaner equipment delivered here to the hospital to go with you when Jessica is discharged. Unfortunately, the biggest holdup right now is the home health piece. They may not have anyone out until the end of next week."

"What does that mean?" I look at Jodie and then Dr. Davidson and back to Jodie. "Does that mean we're here for another week?"

"Well, not necessarily," Dr. Davidson answers quickly. "We believe you and Jesse will be able to provide for Jessica's needs before home health is in place, but there is one more thing that needs to happen before we are comfortable releasing you."

"Which is?"

"One of the biggest indicators we look for in the recovery of a brain injury patient is how well the brain can regulate the blood pressure and heart rate. Right now, Jessica is still on a beta blocker called propranolol that is helping her with this."

"Okay." I'm following him so far.

"We are currently working to wean her off this medication and have, in fact, been pretty aggressive with it. Jessica has been handling it well. However, we are not comfortable having her leave without home health in place, because she will not be monitored while being weaned off the propranolol."

"Well, how much does a blood pressure machine cost? We can buy one if it means that we can monitor her ourselves."

"But what would you do with the information?" Dr. Davidson doesn't wait for me to answer and continues with their plan, which they have probably concocted to determine exactly how many times they can make me cry. "We will continue to wean her off the propranolol. Under our current plan, she will be completely weaned by Saturday. We would like to monitor her for twenty-four hours without the medication and then set you free on Monday morning."

I blink at him a few times, and my shoulders slump. I am racking my brain to find a way of getting out of here tomorrow, but squeezing twelve years of medical education into the next twelve hours so I can properly monitor Jessica as she's weaned off the propranolol is not possible. "Okay."

"Okay?" Dr. Gerritz asks, clearly wondering what my game is.

"Okay." I smile at him. "It's disappointing, but it's a concrete plan. The most concrete answer we've been given in the past seven weeks. So, okay."

Jesse leans back in his chair. "Okay."

"Okay." Jodie hops up. "Then I will look into the status of these items and will be by later with a mountain of paperwork for you to fill out.

"You know where to find me," I tell her. "I'll be pouting and sulking in our room."

She laughs. Without another word, she is dialing her phone. Everyone else pushes their chairs back and collects their belongings.

We shake hands and thank everyone before heading out the door ourselves.

"Are you okay?" Jesse asks as he puts his arm around me again.

I lean into him. "No. I'm really not. As safe as I feel within these hospital walls, I was really looking forward to getting out of here tomorrow."

"Monday isn't bad." He pulls me close and gives me a hug.

"I know."

I'm not okay.

VARIATION UN

Let her sleep, for when she wakes she will move mountains.
Napoléon Bonaparte

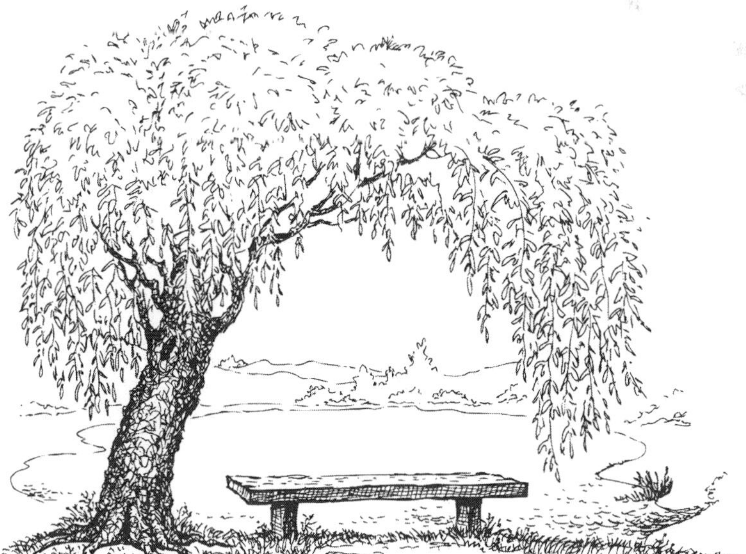

CHAPTER TWENTY

Nothing is Ever Absolutely So

Another four nights in the hospital, another four nights with crappy sleeping arrangements, another four nights away from my husband seems to be too much, and I find myself needing to concentrate on putting one foot in front of the other.

"Just keep your eye on the prize," Jesse tells me. "Monday isn't that far off in the grand scheme of things, especially given all we've been through to this point."

I know he's right. It shouldn't be this big a deal.

But it is. I'm not okay with it.

We reach the room, and I kiss him goodbye before sitting down, feeling defeated. I stare out the window for a little bit, noticing a pair of trees in the distance whose branches form a heart. I take a deep breath and send up a prayer of *Gratitude* to The Universe and my Angels for this simple message.

I turn toward Jessica and begin grounding myself for more meditative healing.

"So, it looks like we're here until Monday. They need to wean you off one more medication, and then we'll get to go home. I can't wait for you to be able to see your Sugar dog and all of our kitties." I remind her not only of the pets waiting for her but the special places in her room, her toys, her clothes, and the layout of our house, trying to give her a jump start on remembering all of it.

Eventually, I stand up and move behind her, pushing the bed

away from the wall so I can place my hands at her crown chakra, calling in the healing energy again.

"Your only job is to remember all of the love, energy, prayers, and light that are still flowing your way. Imagine that I'm pulling it toward you. It is surrounding you and coursing through your whole body, beginning and ending in your beautiful brain. This energy will help your brain reconnect everything that is out of whack.

"Remember that you are the boss of your brain. You get to tell it how much you want to recover. We all believe in you and believe you will be well, but it is most important for you to believe in yourself. Tell your brain what to do, and come back to us."

My voice cracks on this last bit, and I close my eyes and concentrate on keeping my voice steady. "Just come back to us, baby," I whisper as the tears start falling.

After I finish my meditation, I find the lotion and go through our massage routine while singing to her all the songs I've sung to her a million times before. This does nothing to help slow my tears, but I can't seem to stop myself. I cry through "You Are My Sunshine" and weep through "You Gotta Be." By the time I make it through "Everything Possible," I am on the edge of a full-blown breakdown.

"You can dream all the day, never reaching the end of everything possible for you." This line puts me over the edge, and I fall into the chair next to Jessica and sob into her sheets.

I feel a little pathetic.

I feel like I have transcended reality and entered a daytime soap opera.

SCENE: Distraught mother, daughter in coma. Mother clutches daughter's hand, pleading with her to wake up. Mother cries, begs, promises the world, and squeezes daughter's hand. Daughter's eyes flutter. Daughter whispers weakly, "Mommy?"

When will I have my Hollywood moment?

The door to Jessica's room opens, and Amy, the nurse for the night shift, enters.

"Good evening, lad—Oh. Jolene, are you okay?"

I try to wipe my tears and calm my breathing as Amy quickly checks Jessica's vital signs and offers me comfort.

"Can I do anything?"

All I can do is shake my head.

"Can I give you a hug?"

Shaking my head even harder, I bury my face in both hands. I can't explain how a hug would make it worse. So close to the edge of no return, I'm desperate to gain control of my emotions. Human kindness and contact will push me too far in the wrong direction.

As Amy does her evening assessment of Jessica, I work on breathing easier. Amy starts Jessica's feed running and takes care of making her more comfortable. I don't help this time, curling up in my chair instead, whimpering and wiping the tears away as they continue to fall.

"Are you sure there isn't anything I can do? Do you need clean linens? Pillows? Water?"

I decline once again and finally find my voice. "I'm sure, thank you. I'm so sorry you have to deal with me like this."

"Please, don't apologize. You know where to find me if you change your mind."

She leaves the room, and I finally get up to wash my face. Evening has descended, and I haven't bothered to turn on the lights in Jessica's room.

I return to my post and lean over Jessica again. "I'm sorry you have to deal with me, too. I should be stronger for you." I pull up her blankets and kiss her forehead. Her eyes reflect a glimmer of understanding…or so it seems. Again. Not wanting to move her from the position Amy has just put her in, I hug her gently.

"It's dark now," I tell her as I pull away. "It's okay to go to sleep."

Almost on cue, her eyes grow heavier.

I transform my chair into a bed yet again and push it as close to Jessica as possible. I lie down facing her and pull out my phone and earphones. I open the Netflix app and start a rerun of *The Office*, hoping the familiarity will help me zone out enough to get some sleep tonight.

I take a moment to send a text to Jesse: *I am so sad. I miss my baby.*

CHAPTER TWENTY-ONE

Challenge What the Future Holds

Jessica is destined for great things.

From the moment she was conceived, there hasn't been any doubt she is meant to be here on Earth to inspire and change the world.

Despite my being on birth control, Jessica's soul fought her way through, as if mocking the ability of a little pill to thwart the plans we dreamt up.

It was a relatively easy pregnancy, with the only problems arising when I inched closer and closer to my due date. My kidneys threw off increasing levels of protein, but the doctors couldn't find any medical proof of preeclampsia.

The ultrasound performed the day before Jessica's birth scared my body into labor. After forty-five minutes of poking and prodding, the inexperienced tech was unable to determine the position of my baby and declared I would need a C-section "probably immediately." She sent the message to my doctor and scheduled my appointment for the next day.

I never made it to the appointment, as my labor started the same night. Unfortunately, this being my first pregnancy, I didn't realize my back pain was a sign of Jessica's imminent arrival. Instead, I feared something had finally gone very wrong with my kidneys.

Throughout the night, I found relief by taking a series of showers. When I finally spoke to my doctor in the morning, she sounded alarmed that with my "obvious" symptoms, I wasn't already at the hospital.

An hour later, I was in the bathroom of the labor and delivery wing, where my precious girl would make her appearance, when my water conveniently broke into the toilet bowl.

"Okay, honey. I heard that," the nurse called through the door. Come lie down so I can check your progress."

Trying to limit the amount of graphic details, I tried to alert the nurse to my concerns. "I still feel like... something is coming out."

She threw the door open and rushed over to me with one of the big blue pads they sometimes use on the table at visits with a doctor. "Here, let's just put this between your legs."

We clumsily fashioned the pad like a diaper, and I made my way to the bed, climbing up awkwardly, not understanding the alien sensations my body was experiencing.

"Okay, go ahead and lie back," the nurse instructed. I did so, trying to relax.

"All right, you're dilated to ten, but we have a foot. That's what you were feeling."

"A what?"

She didn't answer me. Instead, she picked up the room phone and began to bark orders into it. Magically, two more nurses joined her in the room and they started scribbling on their charts, unhooking the bed from the wall and pushing me through the door.

"What's happening? Where are we going?"

"Your baby's foot is coming out; we need to take you in for an emergency C-section."

"But I don't want a C-section. I want to have natural labor."

"I'm sorry, but you no longer have that option. Your baby is kicking her way into the world."

"Jolene?"

"Where are we going?" I ask stupidly, bolting upright in my chair.

"What? Nowhere. You were dreaming." Amy is by my side. "I'm

so sorry to have to wake you, but I need to ask you about Jessica's medicine. I took her blood pressure, and it's too low to give her the propranolol."

I check the time on my phone, trying to shake off the dream state that is swirling around me. It's midnight.

"They are weaning her off the propranolol," I mumble while rubbing my eyes and trying to wake up enough to understand what Amy needs from me. "It helps with her blood pressure."

"What? No, I know that. If I give her the evening dose of propranolol, it will make her BP dangerously low."

Trying to make sure I understand what Amy is saying, I stare at her for a minute. As the information starts to sink in, I look over at my Fiery Child of Light.

"Don't give it to her."

"That's what I thought. I needed your approval to hold it."

"Yes, please. Skip the evening dose."

"Okay. Again, I'm sorry to have woken you. I'll just change her and then head out."

"I'll help you." I jump up and assist Amy in making Jessica more comfortable. Once done, I accept the hug Amy offered earlier. After I wash my hands, I sit back down to watch Jessica sleep while thinking about my favorite Carl Sagan quote: *Somewhere, something incredible is waiting to be known.*

I bolt awake at 6:00 a.m., determined not to miss a second of the changeover in the nursing shift and the doctors' rounds. I even shower and brush my teeth for the occasion.

Not much has changed, but everything seems different. I'm still so sad to see my baby girl lying in the hospital bed. I'm still drained from yet another crappy night's sleep on a crappy bed. I'm still frustrated and angry about this situation. But it is time to get up, get going, and do the things that need to be done.

Besides, today I have something I haven't had in seven weeks.

A good feeling.

As I throw the used towels and sheets into the linen hamper, I can't fight the smile creeping onto my face.

"What do you think, Jess? Good news today?" I smooch her cheeks and start the rigmarole of getting her changed and comfortable.

Once I'm done placing the last pillow and setting aside her AFOs, I do some quick math in my head and send a text to Jodie:

This is Jolene Lavine. Noooooo pressure at all, but Jessica didn't receive her midnight dose of propranolol. She's been off it for fourteen hours now. If there is ANY way we can still be released today or tomorrow, I would really like to try, please.

Full of nervous energy, I grab my phone and turn on some music to launch our daily routine. Jessica has therapy in a couple of hours. As excited about the day as I am, I want to wait for more answers before I call Jesse.

"Hi, Jolene." Amy has returned. "Laurie will be in soon, but I just wanted to come say bye."

I give Amy another hug and watch as she says goodbye to Jessica. Moments later, Laurie is back.

"So, I hear there is some excitement. You're going home on Monday?" she asks. As she hooks up the BP machine, I can't take my eyes off her hands. She attaches the cuff to Jessica's arm, and I turn to watch the monitor. "Just a little squeeze, Princess."

"So, Monday?" she asks again, pushing the start button.

"Maybe. I'll know more when you tell me how her blood pressure is."

She shoots me a confused look and then reviews her report from Amy. "Oh! They held the midnight dose of propranolol. Her blood pressure was fine without it?"

"Yep." I am clutching the side of the bed now. The monitor beeps, almost on cue. "And now?"

Laurie writes down the number and grins at me. "Golden. We'll skip it again."

I am overwhelmed with emotions and don't know which way to respond first. I settle on a middle ground, letting out a little *whoop* as my eyes fill with tears.

"Okay, so I've already texted Jodie, telling her what's happening and asking if there is any way we can be released today or tomorrow. If it's at all possible, I'd still like to try. Can you let the doctors know what is going on?"

"Of course. I'll send them a message when I'm done here." She rolls up the arm cuff and takes Jessica's pulse. "Her heart rate is a little higher than I'd like, but let me finish assessing her, and I'll check it again." She moves about the room, taking Jessica's vitals, changing the nursing board, and taking inventory of our supplies.

"Maybe if we change her position again, it will help with her heart rate. Her breakfast is running, and she's not quite sitting up high enough."

Once we adjust her bed and add another pillow under her head, her heart rate immediately drops by two points. I make a mental note to pay close attention to this once we're on our own.

"Okay, I'm done here. I'll bring in a couple of supplies and check back in a little bit."

Another time warp whisks me from morning therapy to afternoon therapy. The routine we've built in the hospital over the past seven weeks has become a blur interrupted by meetings with Laurie, Holly the social worker, and Jodie, who hunts me down in one of the therapy sessions to let me know she got my text. She gives me an update regarding the equipment being delivered today, as well as the status of home health.

Hourly checks of Jessica's BP show that it's remaining stable.

The doctors eventually check in, letting us know they will officially discontinue the propranolol.

Jodie eventually reaches home health. They will probably not make it out to our house until the end of next week, but Dr. Davidson and Dr. Gerritz are comfortable with discharging Jessica without home health in place, if we are.

Even though I was pretty sure I knew where Jesse stood on the matter, I call him at work to discuss it anyway and to give him an update on all that has occurred today.

I'm just finishing my report to him when Jodie breezes into the room, wearing a cat-who-ate-the-canary grin.

"Jodie's here. I gotta go. I'll call you back."

"Okay. I love you."

"Love you, too."

Dropping the phone onto its base, I turn to Jodie. "What's up?"

"Eleven o'clock in the morning." Her tone is matter of fact.

"Eleven . . ." I let the number hang in the air between us.

"In the morning. 11:00 a.m. You're outta here."

Stunned by this news, I sit motionless. Could this part of our nightmare be coming to an end? Will life be back to normal soon? Will Jessica finally wake up once she is in her own room? So many questions to be answered, and yet the only thing I seem to be capable of is bursting into tears.

"That's all. I'll leave you alone."

I jump up to give her a quick hug, which I am sure is against some sort of hospital policy, but I can't help it. "Thank you, Jodie. I know I have been unbearable the last couple of days. Thank you so much."

She gives me a cursory squeeze in return and then holds me at arm's length. Giving me a serious look, she says, "Don't ever apologize for being an advocate for your child."

All I can manage to do is nod.

Before Jodie is through the door, I take a deep breath and rush over to the bed.

"You did it." Carefully stroking Jessica's still-broken head, I lean in close and whisper, "I am so grateful to you, my little magical girl. Thank you for giving our family this gift. You weaned yourself off that medicine a full day and a half before the doctors wanted you to. Now they're discharging us two days sooner. You are amazing, Jessica. Not even walking or talking yet, and you're pulling these types of tricks out of your sleeve? I can't wait to see what you have in store for us once you're all better."

I gently kiss her cheeks and then pick up the discarded phone to call Jesse and give him the news.

"D5, this is—" He hasn't even finished his greeting before I'm yelling into the phone.

"Tomorrow! We're going home tomorrow!"

CHAPTER TWENTY-TWO

Mama, I'm Coming Home

June 19, 2010

As we prepared to leave the hospital, I couldn't shake the feeling something big had occurred. Believing as I do in the divine guidance of The Universe, I felt Jessica's higher self joined us in the family meeting and understood what she needed to do to save her mom's sanity. It was a gift for her to wean herself off the medication that was keeping us locked in the medical facility.

When Dr. Gerritz and Dr. Davidson come to see us off and discuss discharge plans with us one more time, I notice that Jessica is doing something new again.

The doctors have been concerned about her gaze preference, the tendency she has to look off to the right 99 percent of the time. Despite the doctors testing her eye movements daily, she hasn't consistently crossed midline with her gaze, and they've been worried.

As we sign the discharge paperwork and the doctors write our last prescriptions, I notice Jessica staring at Dr. Gerritz, who is standing on the left side of her bed. I don't want to bring his attention to it, because I don't want to startle Jessica and break her gaze. I softly clear my throat a couple of times and quickly shift my eyes between Dr. Gerritz and Jessica.

He finally catches on, looks down at her, and gasps. "Jessica!"

The spell is broken, and her gaze shifts to the right again, but Dr. Gerritz grabs her hand and says, "Good job!"

"She was actually staring at you for quite a while," I tell him. "I'm glad I got to witness that before she left. It's very encouraging!"

We finish the discharge paperwork, and Jesse loads the car, leaving me free to roll with the EMTs as they whisk Jessica through the halls and into the elevator to reach the ambulance bay for the ride home.

During the brief moment we're outside before being loaded into the ambulance, I watch Jessica take a deep breath and close her eyes, soaking in the sun that she hasn't felt on her face for seven weeks.

The paramedics let me ride in the back of the ambulance with Jessica, and I enjoy the ride home, especially since Jessica is very relaxed and not at all worked up, as I feared she might be.

When the EMTs push her through the front door of our house, I sense her spirit lighten. There is more than a flicker of understanding in her eyes, and I lean over to brush back her hair and kiss her cheek. "Does it make more sense now?"

The EMTs maneuver the gurney to her bedroom. They transfer her into the hospital bed Jesse set up earlier in the week. As they leave, I almost feel I should tip them for their service, as if to say, "Thanks for the special delivery."

It's just the two of us in the house, so I pull the desk chair to the side of her bed and begin chatting away, as usual. "I know it's a little different than you remember. Dad cleared out some of your stuff to make space for the special bed and the IV pole. We left your pictures and tried to keep as much of your decorating as possible. I hope you remember your room... the library theme you chose because you love to read so much. Your stuffed animals are here in your closet, and, look, there's Nancy."

As I babble on about all the special touches and the things we had done together to decorate the space and make it her own sanctuary, the animals begin to wander in.

Sugar, the dog, comes to sniff me and wag her butt and then investigates Jessica in the bed, licking her hand gently. Bijhu, our eight-year-old Himalayan, wastes no time in jumping onto the bed, which elicits a sound from Jessica I haven't heard in seven weeks. Breathy and guttural, the sound is as close to a laugh as we're going to get, I think.

The other cats wander in and take their places near Jessica. George jumps up on the windowsill, while Jed and Hexe curl up under the bed.

I take Nancy, the snake, out of her tank so Jessica can see her up close. As Nancy tries to slither under the covers, Jessica's breath comes faster and becomes throaty again. It will take a while for me to appreciate this new laugh of hers.

The pieces that don't quite fit in this ten-year-old's bedroom are the boxes of supplies that have been delivered and stacked in the corner. I put Nancy back in her tank and then sit on the floor in front of Jessica's bookcase. Books and art supplies are moved to the floor to make room for multiple cans of Pediasure, which is Jessica's diet now. I stack them neatly on the shelves. As the boxes are emptied of cans, I refill them with the dusty books and art supplies and add them to the boxes already in the closet.

"It's been a big day. Why don't you try to rest a bit. I'm going to check out the house." The only indication that Jessica understands and agrees is the glimmer in her eye and the fact that she closes her eyes.

I pull the curtains closed and walk quietly through the door, leaving it cracked in case she... We'll have our Hollywood moment yet.

Our house is foreign to me now, as other hands have kept it cleaned and organized. I'm struck once more by the vast amounts of space.

In the kitchen, I rifle through the piles of mail on the counter. After separating out the junk mail, tearing off address labels, and starting a shred pile, I simply stare at the stack of bills. I can't bring myself to open them yet.

A hard knock startles me, and Sugar barks. I open the front door to see our good friend Jeff with flowers in one hand and a measuring tape in the other. "Hey."

"What are you doing here?"

"Bringing you these." He sets the flowers on the table and grabs me into a tight hug. I cling to him, willing myself not to crumble completely. "And I need to take measurements for the ramps."

Jeff owns a handyman business called Sunshine Services. He offered to do any renovations we need to make our transition to home easier.

"You don't have to do that today!"

"Shh." He waves me away and starts working. I put the flowers in a vase and continue sorting the mail until another knock has Sugar barking again.

I shush her and open the door. This time it's Kari and Hannah. Hannah is holding a "Welcome Home" balloon for Jessica and a shopping bag, while Kari carries a big brown seat and a soda. A large piece of white equipment sits behind her.

"Hey, ladies," I say in greeting. When they step inside, Kari sets down what I now see is a car seat that will be big enough to stabilize Jessica on the way to doctor's appointments. Together, we grab the larger piece of equipment from the alcove and pull it inside.

"Hi, honey!" Kari pulls me into a hug that rivals the tightness of Jeff's moments earlier. I'm not quite as successful at holding back my tears this time, and I wipe my eyes as I step away from her and kiss Hannah on the head.

"Okay, I'm done." Jeff returns from the garage, gives me another hug, and leaves before I can introduce him to Kari, who is busy pulling lunch from the shopping bag Hannah was holding.

I sit at the kitchen table, and Kari sets a soda in front of me.

"How is Miss Jess?" she asks while serving up a salad that looks like water in a desert after the weeks of institutional food I've been living on.

"She's resting. You can go see her if you want."

"In a minute." She and Hannah sit down to share a meal with me, and things almost feel normal. Sitting with my best friend, having lunch in my home.

We talk about the discharge, and I tell her about Jessica crossing midline for Dr. Gerritz and how well she handled the ride home and the transfer to her new bed. I also tell her about Jessica's new laugh. After I've filled her in with all the details, Kari uses Hannah as a model to train me on the car seat and bath equipment.

"Thank you for this. I don't know what I would do without you." I hug her again. "Let's go check on her. I'm sure she would love to see you."

Jesse arrives home after loading up all of our belongings at the hospital and picking up Jocelyn from day camp.

I hear them crashing through the front door and leave Jessica with Kari and Hannah. I stand in the hall, watching Jocelyn dance around the living room while Jesse sets bags and medical supplies on the table. He looks at me, and I hold my finger to my lips, wanting to watch Jocelyn spin again. He smiles and heads back to the car for the rest of the supplies.

After a few moments, I can't resist the urge to have my youngest girl in my arms, and I step forward. "Jocelyn."

She stops and whips around and then cocks her head at me. "Mama?" she asks, clearly confused about me being here rather than on the seventh floor in the big building, an agonizing forty-minute drive away.

"Hi, baby." I kneel down and hold my arms out. She throws herself into me, and I hold on for dear life. "Hi, baby," I whisper into her hair.

For the rest of the evening, the five of us float in and out of Jessica's bedroom. We chat with and around her, dance silly dances, and sing songs for her. We leave her to rest when her eyes seem droopy, and I take these moments to settle in more, cleaning the house, organizing our new life in closets and drawers, and taking a long shower to clean off the scent of the hospital.

Kari, Hannah, and I leave for a while to go to Target, which had been my plan from the moment we learned we were coming home. I knew we would need to settle in and establish a routine, but I also wanted to build time into the day to do something normal.

Shopping at my favorite store with my best friend and niece, chatting about everyday occurrences rather than medical processes, and trying to laugh again seem like a good way to capture a bit of normal before heading home again.

It's late by the time we return, and I hug and kiss Kari and Hannah goodbye before peeking in on Jessica.

She is sleeping, but when I hold her hand, her eyes flutter open a little, and she squeezes *my* hand. I feel like this must be reflexes, but my heart soars with happiness anyway, hoping she knows I'm here and is glad to have me home.

I watch her until I think she's asleep again, and then I slip out into the hall, wishing her the sweetest of dreams.

CHAPTER TWENTY-THREE

Better Left to Chance

It feels good to be home, not just for what it means for Jessica but for all of us as a family. No more driving to and from, no more packing clothes in and out, no more fast food or cafeteria food, and no more missing my husband and Jocelyn so much I can hardly see straight.

It feels good to be able to work with Jesse to establish some sort of routine for this stage in Jessica's recovery. We're spending the day rearranging the house, finding places for equipment, and working on a schedule for the coming weeks when I get a text message from Melissa: *You're still coming on Tuesday? Second show?*

Tuesday is Jessica's annual recital, the last one she would have performed with Ms. Melissa and Tricks Dance Company. I was hoping Jessica would be well enough to support her fellow teammates, but it looks like it will just be me attending the show.

Of course I am.

When we enrolled Jessica in a Fairytale Ballet class seven years ago, I don't know what we expected. We wanted to get her into some sort of activity to make friends, get some exercise, and learn new skills, but I didn't know how much it would change our lives.

Jessica was three years old when she started dance. We didn't know anything about Tricks or their instructors, so I took the schedule they gave us and drove Jessica to class on Saturdays at 9:00 a.m.

The class picture Jessica has from her first year with Melissa is still sitting on the dance shelf in her room. We've stayed in contact with the families of three of the other four girls who shared the class with Jessica. Melissa was Jessica's instructor throughout our entire time at Tricks, adding her to the performance team when Jessica was six years old.

Without knowing what we were looking for at the time, we got exactly what we needed. Yes, Jessica learned to dance, and she learned it pretty well. She wasn't always the most decorated member of the team; sure, she loved to dance, but it wasn't her passion. She wanted to go out there, be on stage, and have fun. She didn't care about being perfect. She just wanted to shake her groove thing.

We came to learn, know, and live that choreography was not the only part of dance anyway. Bench Time was something I looked forward to each and every week. There were some years that we were at Tricks four or five days a week, and I would joke with the office staff about having them build a room for me out back just to make things easier.

Chatting with other Dance Moms and laughing, arguing, and being extremely catty at times were the highlights of my week. Things aren't always easy or smooth when dealing with so many headstrong women and their daughters, but in the end, I think a very real and true bond developed for most of us.

Jessica never wanted to miss class, because she never wanted to miss seeing her friends, which often got her in trouble since she could be talkative and argumentative with Melissa. Of course, Melissa knew she always had carte blanche to discipline Jessica.

I don't bestow that authority lightly, but trusting Melissa was a no brainer. She's a woman who manages all of the headstrong Dance Moms, makes children fall in love with her at the drop of a hat, and handles crises in her personal and professional life with class. I have loved getting to know her over the years, and seeing the effect she has on all of the dancers who walk through her door is nothing short of magical.

Especially my little dancer.

The small responses Melissa has been able to elicit from Jessica since the time of the accident have simply proven what I have always believed to be true. Melissa is a powerhouse and an incredibly positive force in my daughter's life.

Throughout this horrible experience, our time with the Company is what I miss the most. So, yes. Taking the time to attend the final dance recital that Melissa will be a part of at Tricks is an easy decision.

Or so I thought.

Why did I think it would be so easy to do this?

I close my car door and begin walking slowly toward the theater at Folsom High School but stop in my tracks at the sight of two Company families. One past and one present.

I can't talk to them yet. I'll just go to the back entrance.

I change my course, but it's no use. Jody, another teacher for the Company, is there with her husband and their daughter London. I'm unable to slip inside unnoticed. But as I'm greeting Jody and her family, the Dance Moms and their girls join us, and it's over before it starts.

They take me in through the front entrance, and I feel like I'm home again, hugging each of the moms and tearing up at the sight of the current dancers, made up and ready to perform. My heart expands when I see the past Company members manning a table covered with homemade jewelry and hair clips they've made to sell in support of Jessica.

"You need to sit down," Barb tells me, and I realize I must look as overwhelmed as I feel. I let her lead me into the theater and to the front row.

"You don't have to stay with me," I tell her when she sits next to me.

"Don't be ridiculous. I wanted to talk to you anyway. I'd like to throw a fundraiser for Jessica and your family, to help with your medical expenses."

Her words barely register with me, as the theater fills and memories of seven years of recitals and *The Littlest Nutcracker* holiday shows play in my head.

"Jolene?" Barb places her hand on my arm as I watch a line of ballerinas from the class before Jessica's Friday ballet class climb the stairs and disappear backstage, followed by Brian, the videographer.

"Oh, Brian. He always made sure to put Jessica in the beginning montage of the recital DVDs."

Barb squeezes my arm gently, looks at the stage, and then makes eye contact with me. "Jolene? Take a deep breath."

I close my eyes and do as she says, blocking out the sounds of giggling girls, chattering parents, and teachers calling instructions to one another. I try to block out visions of the chaos in the rooms backstage, where the Dance Company girls have set up shop. Moms trying to find the best angle to take pictures of ballerinas doing their makeup in the big lighted mirrors, hanging from the costume racks and piling themselves on top of one another in tangles of leotards, tutus, and pointe shoes.

"I'm okay," I whisper unconvincingly and look at her again. "Fundraiser? Like a bake sale or something?"

She looks confused and then smiles softly as the lights start flashing. "Yeah, something like that. We'll talk about it later."

The moment the show begins, I'm grateful Barb had the foresight to sit with me. I grab her hand when the dance director talks about Jessica's accident and the love and prayers everyone is sending to her. I don't let go through the numbers I've watched in rehearsal all year. I hang on through Melissa dancing to "Somewhere Over the Rainbow" for Jessica and then blowing kisses to me and giving me a small bluebird before she leaves the stage. I grip her hand tight during the final performance by the Company girls, all of them wearing purple bracelets in honor of Jessica.

When the lights come up and people exit the theatre, we hang back in our seats, and I attempt to compose myself.

"That was beautiful," Barb says softly.

"It was. I knew this was going to be emotional; I just didn't think it all the way through. This was too much. I know everyone is pulling for Jessica, but to be here in the midst of all this love? It's overwhelming. Thank you for sitting with me. I can't believe this is over. This is it."

CHAPTER TWENTY-FOUR

Don't Blink

I'm feeling overwhelmed and wiped out, in both good and bad ways. Jessica is progressing so fast now that I feel I am missing the small bits and pieces of her recovery. She changes so quickly from day to day, and I don't have enough time to update the Facebook page I created to document her journey. When people come to visit Jessica, they are often surprised that she is doing better than they expected.

BLINK

It is becoming much easier to communicate with Jessica. Not only is she beginning to use her hands to indicate yes and no, but we are able to discern from her facial expressions what she is and isn't okay with. This has helped alleviate some stress from our day.

BLINK

"Jessica, you have a visitor." My friend Kelly has been asking when her son, Collin, can visit. Collin and Jessica have been friends since preschool days. They have a very sweet friendship, and I have been hesitant to let him visit because I've been hoping for further recovery before he sees Jessica. I neglected to think about the healing power a visit from him might wield.

Jessica looks at Collin as he walks through the door, and I am astonished to see her laughing and trying to vocalize while attempting to hoist herself off the bed. She lifts her bottom and moves her legs up and down. She is even able to lift her shoulders and torso higher than we've seen her do in the past.

"Hi, Jessica." Collin's face breaks into a huge, toothy grin, and he moves toward her. Jessica continues to laugh and try to talk to her best buddy.

I shouldn't have waited so long.

BLINK

I'm sitting in my usual place at Jessica's desk while she rests after her morning wheelchair time. Her lunch is running through the pump.

I turn on the TV and scroll through the DVR recordings to find something to watch while checking email and paying bills. I start an episode of *So You Think You Can Dance*, adjust the volume to a low level, and turn my attention to the computer, punching in logins, passwords, and financial information.

An hour later, the food pump alerts me to the completion of the first cycle. I get up to add water to the second cycle and notice that Jessica is looking at the TV. Normally, her head pulls to the left due to the tone and spasticity caused by the injury. Apparently, her favorite TV show is motivation enough for her to work on crossing midline.

BLINK

"Jessica, can you choose the pink marker?"

I hold a purple marker in my left hand and a pink marker in my right. I lean toward her, trying to hold the markers at the same distance and height so as not to influence her.

It takes her a minute to conjure up the strength, but eventually she thrusts her left arm forward, knocking the pink marker with her hand.

"Can you choose the card that has the five on it?" Success.

"Which one shows the answer to two plus two?" Success.

"Which card equals three times two?" Success!

I finally pull out the yes and no cards and ask her, "Is your name

Nicole?" *No.* "How about Heather?" *No.* "Then it must be Ellie!" *No.* "Jessica?" *YES.*

We have communication!

BLINK

"Jessica, you have a visitor."

It's Melissa this time. I've asked her to come by with the music she uses in ballet class, to test Jessica's muscle memory. I sit at Jessica's desk, tears in my eyes, while the classical music fills Jessica's room.

Melissa begins. "Plié, tendu, dégagé...," and a memory rolls into me suddenly.

Saturday rehearsal before performing at the Harlem Globetrotters game on Monday. Garth Brooks' song If Tomorrow Never Comes *floating through the dance room at the Granite Bay studio. Nineteen girls in fluorescent hot pink stand at the barre, all moving in unison as Melissa walks among them.*

Melissa reaches out to lift Jessica's leg, moving it through the air, and calls out the moves once more. "Relevé, frappé..."

BLINK

"Who's there?" I shoot up in bed, reaching for Jesse, who lifts his head to listen.

CLANK, followed by a soft giggle.

Jesse sits up now. "What is that?" We are stone still, trying to decipher the noise in the otherwise quiet house.

CLANK. More giggles.

"Is someone here?" I whisper in his ear.

"Stay here. Sugar, come." Sugar is up instantly, following Jesse out of the bedroom.

CLANK. Giggle.

I watch Jesse turn down the hall and then hear him carefully open Jocelyn's bedroom door. He closes it seconds later.

CLANK. Laughter.

That can't be, I think to myself, moving the covers, jumping up, and rushing through the door. Jesse meets me at the door of Jessica's bedroom, and we stand and listen for a moment.

CLANK. Laughter.

"What the...?" He reaches out and opens the door, and we find Jessica wide awake, her leg, splinted in the heavy and clunky AFO, resting on the metal rail of her hospital bed. As we watch, she lifts her leg to bang the AFO on the metal rail and then dissolves into a fit of laughter.

Jesse and I look at one another, smiles creeping onto our faces. "She's regaining control," I whisper to him.

BLINK

"I am so tired," I whine to Jesse as we share a rare moment in the bathroom, him in the shower and me at the sink, preparing for our day.

"Yeah?" He calls over the water.

"It's all changing so fast."

BLINK

"Ahh."

I look up from my sentry post at the desk to see Jessica grinning at me.

"Ahh?" I whisper back to her.

"Ahhhhhh," she repeats, starting to giggle. I get up and move closer.

"Ahhhhh!" I raise the volume just a bit.

"Ahhhhhh!" She sees my raise, and her face squishes up in silent laughter. I can't keep a straight face and start giggling at her. At me. At *us.*

"Ahhhhhhh!" We both yell at one another and lose ourselves in laughter.

BLINK

We're sitting in the waiting room of the ER, waiting to get Jessica's throat checked. Our yelling matches allowed me to see that one of her tonsils is swollen. She also seems to have some pain on the left side of her neck.

"Hic." I shift my attention from the TV mounted on the wall to where Jessica sits in her wheelchair.

"What was that?" I ask her.

"Hic."

"Is this the first time she's had the hiccups since her accident?" I ask Jesse, who is holding a sleeping Jocelyn in the chair next to me.

"I hadn't thought about it, but I think so."

"Hic."

"Weird little milestone."

BLINK

We're home from the ER, and Jessica is lying down, lights are out, and we're settling in for the night.

"Achoo!" she says, followed by a giggle.

"Salud!" I whisper to her and believe it's love. I cherish the little pieces I never thought to miss.

BLINK

"So fast," he says as he steps from the shower and towels off.

"Laughing, moving...even the pain in her neck allow us to see how she responds to the pain and our attempts to comfort her."

"Yeah, she was definitely enjoying the massage you gave her yesterday to help with the pain."

"Yeah. It's clear. She's here with us. She understands exactly what is going on."

"Yeah, she does."

"Even though some parts of her recovery are still difficult, I do feel like changes are taking place. I feel that we're turning a corner. The sparks are finally going off in her brain, and the pieces that were jumbled up are starting to fall into place."

He finishes toweling off and grabs his deodorant from the drawer. "Well, she's probably done with being cooped up and having her movements restricted."

"True." The reflected dimensions in the mirror mesmerize me as I tick tasks off on my fingers. "Medication, therapy, our morning or evening meditations, my showerfestation—"

"You lost me," he calls from the closet attached to the bathroom. "Showerfes . . . what?"

"I do a meditation in the shower every day. I call it showerfestation."

He emerges from the closet and gives me a quick peck on the lips. "I love you."

"Are you mocking me?"

"Not at all."

"You know it's not just me. Every day I still receive messages about the love, energy, and prayers being sent. Any or all of it is helping to bring her back. Mojo, juju, hocus pocus, or people dancing around the campfires shaking tambourines."

He's sitting now, tying his shoes. "Oh, come on. You know what it is."

I lean against the wall, confused by his certainty. "Um. No?"

"Let's see, you've done all the foofoo stuff, you've cried, you've begged, you've even used logic to explain to her how her brain can heal itself. What haven't you mentioned?"

I shake my head and shrug.

He takes me by the shoulders. "The bribes, honey."

"The bribes!"

"What have you promised her?"

"Well, my old laptop; an iPhone; trips to New York, Paris, and

Disney World; the Harry Potter Experience; Disneyland; Monterey; a shopping spree at Justice, Old Navy, and Target; a DS with unlimited games." I pause to look at him. "I hope she forgets about that one. And a full collection of Webkinz."

"Right. You see? I know why she's progressing so quickly now."

I nod and return to the bathroom to finish dressing. "She's coming to collect."

BLINK

The in-home therapists have recommended we get Jessica into inpatient therapy.

It's time.

BLINK

"Lance asked me today what kind of insurance I wanted." Jesse is on his lunch break at work and has called to check in. He drops this piece of news on me, and I can only stare at the desk, not understanding his statement.

"What?"

"Our open enrollment is here. If we want to switch insurance, now's the time."

"Are you kidding me?" I jump from my seat and begin pacing the small space in Jessica's room. I can hardly contain my excitement. I notice that she follows me with her eyes. I stop at the foot of the bed, smiling at her and trying not to jump out of my skin.

"Yeah. He has information for a couple of different options and is asking for my input."

"Whatever we can do to get in the UC Davis Health System. Whatever it will take to make that work. Yes, yes! Oh, my gosh. I could kiss Lance right now! Does he realize he's my hero?"

"I'd prefer you didn't, and I don't know if he realizes. I'll let him know."

BLINK

It's amazing how the changes in our circumstances can change our perspective on what we once thought of as a problem.

I haven't slept well since the day of the accident. While the insomnia has been a hassle, tonight my insomnia is caused by *good* possibilities rather than tragic events. I'm so excited about the new opportunities a new insurance plan will bring to Jessica's care.

Also, after I helped her get ready for sleep, she had trouble relaxing, so I repositioned her and eventually took off her AFOs, figuring a break for one night wouldn't hurt. When she fell asleep, she had rolled onto her side, and her right leg was bent up on her left leg. Without the AFOs on, she is able to sleep like a normal little kid.

It does my heart good.

BLINK

"Did she just say 'Mom'?" Jesse asks me as we all hang out in Jessica's room, folding laundry, reading, and watching Jocelyn dance.

"Don't get my hopes up," I tell him with a soft smile.

"Mah?" From the bed.

"Pretty sure that's 'Mom,'" Jesse insists while Jessica grins at me. I can barely breathe.

BLINK

"Are you excited for school to start?" I ask Mallory, one of Jessica's friends from Brighton. She and her mom, Shannon, have come to visit, and we're painting the girls' nails while chatting.

"Yeah," Mallory replies.

Jessica's face twists into a grimace, and she begins to cry.

"What is it, Baby Girl?" I put the nail polish on the side table and begin my routine check of Jessica's body, looking for pinches, creases, bad positioning, or anything that may be causing her pain.

She shakes her head, and I think about our conversation while shifting her position just a bit.

"Oh, are you sad because we were talking about going back to school?"

Jessica nods.

"Oh, sweetheart. You will return to school soon. Even if you were all better and able to go to school, too, there are still activities you would miss out on. We can't do everything all of the time, and right now your job is bigger than going to school. Your homework is to work on getting better."

BLINK

"I've noticed you working on your right hand more, Jess." This week she grabbed for a stuffed animal, and she held my arm when I changed and repositioned her. I've also seen her fiddle with her clothes.

Proving me right, she wiggles her fingers at me. I pull the chair over and sit down so I'm at her level. I grab my phone from my pocket and open the keypad.

"Can you touch the number seven?" I ask her. She slowly lifts her arm and hits the keypad with her hand lightly.

"Great job. Now we just need to work on your fine motor, huh?" I try not to let my excitement overwhelm her as I visualize her having control over her hands and fingers. Fine motor control would allow her to use a speech device. I don't know how I'm holding back my tears of joy.

BLINK

Our new insurance is finally in place. I spend the morning making calls to establish Jessica with a new primary care physician, get on the schedule with Dr. Manhart, and, most importantly, talk to neurosurgery about having Jessica's head put back together. These steps need to be taken before we can pursue inpatient therapy. My body hums in a constant state of excitement over this next step.

By the end of the week, the phone rings. Despite not recognizing the 734 prefix on caller ID, something tells me to answer anyway. A recorded voice comes on the phone: "This is the UC Davis Medical Health Care System. Jessica Lavine has an appointment with Dr. Manhart—"

"Yes, she does!" I yell, as the automated voice drones on with the details.

The ball is rolling.

BLINK

CHAPTER TWENTY-FIVE

Crawling Down the Avenue

"I think I need to create some kind of routine." Jesse and I are lounging in bed in the early morning hours, speaking quietly over the sleeping toddler who snores between us.

"What kind of routine?" He holds my hand, tracing it with his thumb.

"I don't know. A schedule for therapy and basic care for Jess balanced with something more normal, like cleaning or organizing. Some sort of therapy and cleaning routine to help the days go faster. I'm so impatient for her head to be put back together."

"That sounds like a good plan."

"Yeah. It will give me a chance to contribute to the upkeep of the house and keep me from making our whole day about therapy and rehab."

"It'll also give her a chance to see more day-to-day stuff, as Faye suggested before we left the hospital in June."

"Right. I forgot about that." I chew on my lip, assembling a schedule in my head. "Yeah, maybe seeing me bustle about the house as I did before will help jog some memories for her."

"Yes, and since you're here with her all day, you need to be able to find a balance between want to's and need to's. I don't want you getting burnt out."

"I agree. It'll also keep me from sitting around willing time to go faster. I hope keeping busy will help the days and weeks fly by."

No matter what else I do, that's all I wish for. All day long.

5:30 a.m.—Administer medications and fluids, put on AFOs.

6:00 a.m.—Start feed running from pump. While feed is running (hour and a half), take shower, get dressed, start laundry, check email and Facebook, write an update.

7:30 a.m.—Toileting, take off AFOs, move her to wheelchair, work on speech therapy.

8:30 a.m.—Clean kitchen.

9:00 a.m.—Jessica back to bed, administer meds and fluids, brush teeth, wash face, sponge bath, wash hair (carefully due to missing skull). Change position, toileting, put on AFOs. Lights down for low stimulation while I work on laundry, make phone calls, check email and Facebook.

11:30 a.m.—Change position, toileting, take off AFOs.

12:00 p.m.—Administer fluids and meds, start feed running from pump, lunch for me, straighten house.

1:30 p.m.—Change position, toileting, put on AFOs.

2:00 p.m.—Therapies.

3:30 p.m.—Toileting, take off AFOs, into wheelchair, go outside for a dose of sunshine.

4:30 p.m.—Administer fluids.

5:30 p.m.—Back to bed, toileting, put on AFOs. Start dinner, Jesse and Jocelyn come home. Family bonding in Jessica's room. Reading, music, movie, talking.

6:00 p.m.—Administer meds, start feed running, dinnertime.

7:30 p.m.—Change position, toileting, take off AFOs, lights down, candles lit, low stimulation, quiet time in house.

9:00 p.m.—Administer medications and fluids.

9:30 p.m.—Change position, toileting, put on AFOs, reading, soft music, meditation, energy work.

10:30 p.m.—Bedtime.

The worst feeling in the world is when your child is screaming in pain, and you can't do a damn thing to fix it.

The routine we have been settling into has been thrown off this week due to the discomfort Jessica is experiencing in the evening hours. She has begun screaming, yelling, and crying for hours each night.

When it first happened, Jesse and I spent the entire evening searching for the source of what we perceived to be Jessica's pain. We addressed everything we could think of, from her G-tube site leaking to the muscle tension in her neck. We tried to communicate with her to find out if she had an itch or a cramp somewhere, but those attempts failed, drowned out by the storm of emotions coursing through her.

We tried changing her body position, changing the position of the bed, getting her into her wheelchair, offering her a movie. We took her outside, gave her a bath, and even stretched her out and meditated with her on the therapy mat in the living room.

Nothing seemed to work, but after we laid her down again and turned the radio on low, she started to calm down.

When it happened the following night, Jesse hadn't gotten home from work yet, so I stayed with Jessica in the bedroom and tried to calm her down by meditating with her, seeking comfort with her, and doing my best to reassure her.

The following night, alone again, I tried an even quieter approach and left the room completely. I was mindful of noise, so I didn't do much more than sit on the couch and mess around on my phone. When Jesse and Jocelyn got home, the three of us had a quiet dinner at the table. After about an hour, I checked in on Jess. She was still anxious and uncomfortable but nothing like she'd been the past couple of nights.

I read to Jesse from the computer screen as we check our email at the end of the night. "Maybe it's similar to the 'witching hour' that some babies go through."

"What's that?" He looks up from his computer.

"I was venting on Facebook about Jess's discomfort and our inability to figure out what's going on with her, and Mary suggested the witching hour as an explanation."

He returns to his computer, and his fingers fly across the keys. He pauses at one article and reads it out loud. *Every night, sometime between 4:00 p.m. and 9:00 p.m., nothing you do will satisfy your baby. It's the witching hour.* He looks up and says, "Yeah, that could be it."

"Maybe she just needs an hour or so with absolutely no stimulation in the evenings. We had the best luck tonight. No music, no lights, and me out of the room. The couple of hours before bed were touch and go, but it was easier to make her laugh—"

"Fewer outbursts, too." He takes a drink from the wine glass sitting on his desk.

"Let's try it again tomorrow and see what happens."

"You know, I also wonder if she's just becoming more aware and is getting more emotional about her situation."

The idea of this awareness and my previously independent daughter feeling so trapped immediately chokes me up. "Oh, do you think?"

"It's possible. She could just be shedding tears out of frustration and sadness."

"You may be right. It's very draining." I wipe at my tears as I continue scrolling through my Facebook feed.

"Well, you still handle it like Superwoman."

I scoff. "Sometimes. Mostly, I feel that I'm screwing up Jessica's chances at recovery, damaging Jocelyn's chances of growing up in a normal household, and destroying our marriage, all in one fell swoop."

"Oh, honey. You are not."

"You're sweet." I smile at him and begin sorting the mail from the day. "But you can't deny I've been completely irritable with you this week."

"True, but I just thought you were PMSing or something."

My eyebrows shoot up, and I try to glare at him. "Did you really just say that?"

He gets up and kisses me on the head and starts getting into his pajamas. "Yes, but you know I'm joking. It's a tough situation; you're allowed a little bit of irritability."

"Pshaw. Don't tell Sabrina that."

"Who?"

"Sabrina Hendricks. You met her last year."

"Okay. Why shouldn't I tell her that?"

"Oh, because according to her, I'm mad about all of the good stuff happening in her life."

He drops his hands to his sides and stares at me. "Are you serious?"

"Yeah." I shut down my computer and begin moving pillows and pulling back the covers. "Then she lectured me, telling me that even though our situation is bad, I shouldn't compare my life to others and think I'm handling more than them."

"Right. That sounds like something you do every day, with all your free time."

"Right? What's even better is that she went on to do exactly that, comparing her life to ours and telling me all the stuff she is handling throughout her day. Her job, her kids, her husband, her family troubles."

"She's obviously very important," he says in a deadpan tone.

"Yeah, I told her I'm handling pretty much all of the same things, in addition to caring for Jessica. Of course, I should have just disengaged."

"Don't stick your hand in the crazy, after all."

"Especially since I was wrong."

"What?" He turns on his side to face me. "What were you wrong about?"

"I'm not doing as much as she is in addition to caring for Jessica. But here's the thing . . . I would gladly take on all the responsibilities she has if it meant Jessica would be well.

"What she listed are tasks I did every day before the accident. I had the same commitments, along with caring for the girls, shuttling Jessica to her activities, volunteering for projects for those activities, taking Jocelyn to playgroup, and working to get a business off the ground."

"You definitely didn't sit around watching movies and eating bonbons."

"Nope. These days, even with the schedule we created, I'm busy with the dishes (if I'm lucky), laundry (if I'm lucky), and dusting and vacuuming (if I'm lucky).

"I'm still caught up in phone calls with The Pit, straightening out the charges before we escaped, as well as all the calls to the new insurance company to set up the necessary services.

"I'm still trying to schedule meetings with Alta about respite care and with the school district for her IEP, not to mention scheduling the therapists and visitors coming and going..."

"Then you get into Jessica's care." He picks up the ball for me. "Medications five or six times a day, body care, repositioning, putting on and taking off the AFOs and hand splints throughout the day, and writing it all down so we have a record for the next doctor's appointment."

"Right. And none of that, not one of those tasks, takes as much energy or is as difficult to perform as what I've had to do this week."

"What's that?"

"Sitting by Jessica's bed, holding her hand, rubbing her head, and whispering comfort in her ear while attempting to meditate, breathe, and simply try anything to help her through the pain and discomfort she was feeling. For an hour and a half. Three nights in a row.

"I've lit candles, meditated, pulled in the energy I know everyone continues to send. I've changed the volume and pitch of my voice, hoping my words will reach her somehow. The words I hope will give her some comfort: 'You are healing; you are safe; you are loved; you are healing.'"

He moves closer to me and begins stroking my hair. "It won't always be like this."

"How do you know? It's maddening that Sabrina thinks she needs to lecture me. I could give a fuck what she has going on in her life. What we have going on is overwhelming and painful. It's the most difficult experience of my life. I don't have the energy to compare my life or what we do to anyone else's experience.

"Everyone has their own pain to deal with, their own crosses to bear. I wouldn't want to trade lives with anyone. I don't know the challenges they face or if I would have the fortitude to face them with as much grace as some people do.

"But I do know this: If it meant Jessica could be up and dancing, walking, talking, and singing her way through life again, I would gladly handle anything *anyone* throws at me. I would happily handle the level of stress and busyness we had in our lives before April if it meant I never again had to hold Jessica's hand while she screams. To never again have to try desperately to convince her that what I say is true: *You are healing.*"

CHAPTER TWENTY-SIX

Feel a Change in Everything

"Okay, Jess, I know your neck is still hurting and you may be a little uncomfortable in your chair while we're here, but let's try to really show Dr. Manhart your stuff." I try to boost Jessica's confidence while Jesse pushes her through the hall that leads directly to the outpatient PM&R Department. "Please try your hardest to respond when he asks you to do something so he can help you continue to get better."

The receptionists at the check-in desk greet Jessica with genuine joy in their voices. "Welcome back, Jessica! It's so good to see you!"

Jessica grins in response.

"Not quite talking yet. Sorry," I tell them. "We have an appointment with Dr. Manhart at 11:30."

"Of course you do. Have a seat, and they'll take you back in a minute."

"Thank you." We barely have time to sit down before a medical assistant is calling us back to take Jessica's vitals.

Once Jessica's weight, BP, and temperature are recorded, the medical assistant asks, "Do you prefer to go back to the lobby, or would you like to wait in the inner office here?"

"Oh, we'll stay in here if that's okay."

"No problem at all." The medical assistant leads us to a room closer to the exam rooms. Jesse positions Jessica's wheelchair at the end of the chairs. I sit next to Jessica and pull out my phone to help her focus on something other than the commotion in this small space.

She is laughing at the SmackTalk app when Holly, the social worker we worked with while we were in the hospital, comes around the corner.

"I thought I recognized that laughter. Hey, Jessica!"

"Holly! Hi!" I stand up to give her a quick hug.

"So you're back, yes?"

"We sure are. Got our insurance changed, and she is all yours now."

"That's great. Let me check if there's a room ready."

"Okay, thanks." I sit on the edge of the seat, trying not to fidget too much.

Jesse grabs my knee to calm my leg, which is bouncing up and down. "Excited?"

"How could you tell?" Grinning at him, I wiggle my toes inside my shoes instead.

Holly returns and says, "Okay, guys, let's go in here." We follow her into the exam room. I expect her to just drop us there and say goodbye, but she follows us in and sits down.

"So, how are things going at home?"

Jesse and I glance at one another, and I take a deep breath. "They're going okay. Some good days; some bad days."

"Are you getting a break at all?" She crosses her legs and opens the folder to take some notes.

"I try. Jesse is so supportive of me going out when he gets home from work or on the weekends."

"No nurse yet?"

"Not yet. Still getting all of the bits settled with the new insurance, and our intake appointment with Alta Regional hasn't happened yet."

"It can take a while, that's for sure. And how are you doing, Jessica?"

Jessica watches Holly's face and grins while Jesse and I fill her in on all of the little pieces of Jessica's progress since being home.

"It sounds like being home has had the desired effect then?" Holly asks.

"It sure has."

"I imagine being home makes it easier for people to visit her, too."

"For the most part, yes. It has definitely been easier for her friends to come visit."

The idea of spending time with her friends causes Jessica to start laughing and moving around in her wheelchair.

"Oh, that got her attention." Holly laughs along with Jessica.

"For sure."

A quick knock echoes through the room, and Dr. Manhart pushes the door open. "Who's making all that noise?"

Holly stands to let Dr. Manhart have the chair and gives my shoulder a quick squeeze. "I'll see you later." She leans down so she is face-to-face with Jessica. "I am so glad you're back with us."

My eyes fill with tears at this as Dr. Manhart signs onto the computer.

"Welcome back," he says. "How are things going with Jessica?"

During the rest of the appointment, I report the changes and progress we've recorded in Jessica's recovery notebook, and Jesse offers the less clinical, more anecdotal, samples of our daily life. We share the progress she's made, our daily schedule, her therapies, the medications the old HMO doctors prescribed for her, the equipment we have... pretty much every aspect of Jessica's care.

He listens to our assessments, notes the items she needs, and explains the changes he would like to make in her treatment. After ordering labs and a bone scan, he writes a prescription for additional pieces of equipment and talks about weaning her off the neurostimulants so he can get a baseline of how responsive she is now.

With the business part of the appointment done, he rolls over to where Jessica sits in her wheelchair. I miss what he says to her, as I'm overwhelmed with emotion at Jessica being back in his care. It is a relief to have her with a doctor who believes in her abilities. A doctor who will not focus only on maintaining the status quo of her recovery but who will figure out how to move her forward.

He asks Jessica to track his finger, which she does, and checks her reflexes, which causes her to laugh out loud.

"Okay, Jessica. I need you to squeeze my fingers, okay?"

I hold my breath, hoping she has enough strength and stamina left at this point to follow his commands.

"Great."

She does.

"That's old stuff. Right, Jess?" I tease her. "Is it too easy?"

"Oh?" Dr. Manhart says. "Show me something new then."

"Well, she might not be able to do this since she's been in the chair for a while today, but this week we've been working on having her move her hand to her chest."

"From her side?" he asks.

"Yes. I straighten her arm at her side and ask her to bring her hand to her chest. The first day I asked her to do this, she could only wiggle her fingers a little bit, but the next day her whole hand tried to move."

At this point, I straighten Jessica's arm out. "Can you move your hand to your chest, honey?" I start to reiterate my warning to Dr. Manhart. "She can't do it yet, but the effort is obv—"

Jessica doesn't give me a chance to finish my warning before she moves her entire forearm toward her chest.

"Whoa! Jessica!" I am laughing and crying while Jesse pats her on the back.

"Good job, honey!"

"Well, she showed you, I guess," Dr. Manhart comments.

"I guess she did. Oh, my goodness. That's the most responsive and purposeful movement she's shown yet."

"Well, that's what we like to see. More stuff like that, Jess, and you'll be ready for inpatient rehab."

My head snaps up. "Yes! When will that be do you think?"

"Well, she still needs to have her head put back together and continue working on this type of thing. The stronger she can get and the more she responds to commands, the more effective inpatient rehab will be for her. It probably won't be for another three to six months, so that neurosurgery has time to fix her head."

My shoulders slump, and he says quickly, "That's a conservative timeline. If she gets in for surgery quicker and has a strong recovery, it could be faster. We just have to wait and see."

My mind races, thinking about all the renovations to our car and home we've been putting off, because we believed she would be better by now. Knowing that she won't even be in rehab for at least another three months makes the decision to convert the van or the bathroom easier.

Dr. Manhart interrupts my thoughts. "I am definitely encouraged by her progress. We'll talk again in three months, if not before then."

He gets up to signal the end of the appointment, and we stand to shake his hand. "Thank you, Dr. Manhart. Thank you so much."

"She's making her way back. See you all soon," he says casually as he gives us our discharge paperwork and leaves the office. Jesse and I just stare at each other.

"She's making her way back." Jesse echoes the prediction, and I'm crying again.

CHAPTER TWENTY-SEVEN

So Hard to Handle

I have stopped and started one hundred emails. I don't know how I am ever going to come back from this.

I type and then stare at the computer screen, hands poised above the keyboard, index fingers tapping the F and J keys. Sara Bareilles' voice flows from my earphones, and tears are streaming down my face. I feel ill-equipped and melodramatic but desperate to send this email to my closest friends, hungry for their words of advice and comfort.

My idle hands find music of their own and add some lyrics to the screen.

Now I done lost the best baby that I ever had…

This song, originally by Joni Mitchell, always gets to me. When I found a cover of it performed by my daughter's favorite female singer, I immediately added it to the ever-growing playlist I created back in May.

I wish I had a river I could skate away on.

That line, more than any other, does little to comfort my broken heart. Before sobs overwhelm me completely, I take a deep breath and type.

My daughter was kicked in the head by a horse.

We are five months out from The Accident, which is how I refer to it when talking about it nowadays, and I am still looking for a less dramatic way of stating what happened.

To simply say, "My daughter was kicked in the head by a horse," sounds dramatic and horrible.

It was.

It was dramatic and horrible.

The accident is much more ambiguous and could have been anything. She could have torn a ligament dancing or broken her leg doing gymnastics. Maybe burned her hand in a campfire or fallen from the bars at school. It could have been anything innocent and simple.

But it wasn't.

My daughter was kicked in the head by a horse.

I don't know how any of us will ever come back from this.

I wish I had a river so long I could teach my feet to fly.

Jesse and I are relaxing on the couch after the girls are in bed.

"I'm wrung out. Things have been going better this week, but even with the schedule to guide me, time is crawling, answers from neurosurgery are slow, and I don't know how to sustain this pace."

"Well," Jesse says, "I was looking at the new policy, and besides getting her head put back together and inpatient therapy, you know what else we can do?"

"What?"

"Hire a nurse."

I sigh and shift my position.

"I know you don't think we—" Jesse starts again.

"I don't think we need to. We shouldn't have to. I'm home all day. I should be able to take care of her myself."

Jesse scoots closer to me and reaches out to run his fingers through my hair. "But you just said…"

"I know. I just need to figure out how to get a break and how to find a way to interact with other people. I'm so isolated right now. Plus, it's weird…"

"What is?"

"Being home is definitely the best therapy for her. She's sitting in her chair longer and longer each day. She focuses more on the TV. She likes it when the radio is on and has been reacting to different songs."

"Oh?"

"Yeah, when we were working on therapy yesterday, she was yelling about it, but as soon as I pointed out the new Sara Bareilles song on the radio, she calmed right down."

"So what's weird then?"

"Sitting in the hospital room with only a couple of reminders of our life together was entirely different from being here. In our own space." I look up at the wall of family photos. Jessica dancing here, the four of us on a sleigh ride there, school pictures, family and friends surrounding us in gales of laughter, and a net of love cast far and wide. "Here in our own space, with our family history surrounding us, it's a constant reminder of how things were. I continually hope, wish, and pray for life to be that way again in the future."

Dear Jessica,

I'm sorry, little girl, but I think I'm breaking down. I've made an appointment with a therapist to get some help coping with the hole I have in my chest after your accident, but this week I just got overwhelmed. I needed to get away.

There is no place I'd rather be than by your side through this ordeal, but being a caregiver is hard work, no matter how much you love the person for whom you are providing care.

And I do love you.

That never changes, but I hope you remember I have always said I want to be as honest with you as possible. I would be lying if I said loving you made all of this easy. It doesn't. In fact, I feel like loving you makes caregiving harder.

Losing the relationship we had before your accident has been tough.

Snuggling with you, laughing with you, joking, talking, singing, and all of our everyday experiences. Surprising you with gifts or trips or even just a toy or a note in your lunch. Girls' day out for nails or dinner…

I can only hope we will experience all of this again, but being without these special times while you're recovering has been hard.

I needed a break. Your dad and I agreed I could get out of town for the weekend. I'm on my way to spend time with friends in Oregon, but I've stopped by the ocean on the way. I wanted to put my feet in the sand and capture some ocean water for you.

Unfortunately, it's too late and cold now to imagine getting out of the car, and the parking lot I'm in doesn't have great beach access.

Instead, I'm sitting in the car with the windows rolled down, feeling the cold wind blow in from the sea and watching the waves roll in. Wading into the water probably wouldn't have been safe anyway, as there are so many waves, and they are crashing fast.

I'm breathing the ocean air deep, asking the Spirits of the Sea to remove this tension and anger within me. I imagine my emotions rolling and crashing like the waves, strong and powerful but resting gently and quietly as they reach the shore.

And you are my shore, Baby Girl. I know I don't always succeed in keeping my emotions gentle and quiet, and I'm sorry for that.

You have always been and always will be the place I come home to. You saved me, sweet girl, and as the waves wash to the shore, may you always feel my love washing over you.

For I do. I love you always and forever. That never ends.

Love,

Mom

People keep telling me to take care of myself, and I'm confused about what more I'm supposed to do.

Most of the time, I think I'm doing okay. I'm handling our days and moving things along. Trying to breathe. To go with the flow. To do what needs to be done.

I care for Jessica 90 percent of the time during the week, only getting an hour or so to sort my own thoughts in the evenings after Jesse gets home or on the weekends when he happily cares for both girls while I do whatever I need to do. Then I scrapbook with friends, get a massage, or even do the mundane and mindless act of grocery shopping.

Most of the time this works. Our new life is not easy, but I feel like I'm getting there. I'm trying to adapt to the circumstances, changes, and challenges. We didn't ask to be put in this situation, and we're simply trying to do the best we can. Usually that effort is good enough for most people.

I make some mistakes, but for the most part, I'm here. Doing what needs to be done, because, really . . . where else would I be?

There are days, however, like the one that happened this week. While Jesse made arrangements for doctors' appointments, therapies, and getting our van converted, someone complained to him, saying, "It's just one thing after another."

One comment is all it takes, and I'm drowning in the numerous mind-numbing, heartbreaking, soul-crushing interactions I've had since Jessica's accident.

Tempers flaring, raw feelings exposed, hurtful and destructive dialogue. Each criticism of how I'm handling this situation, the accusations of taking advantage of people, being told I'm not worth the time or energy it takes to maintain a relationship with me, being thrust aside and written off.

All the things I'm doing right for Jessica are muffled by the roar of the machine gun in my head. The rapid fire of people who stand in line wasting their time just to hate me.

I want someone to be on my side. I want to be given the benefit of the doubt, as I give it to others. Instead, so many relationships have ended because of assumptions and arrogance. I wonder what it would feel like to have someone consider me worth the effort that goes into truly moving beyond conflict, settling into forgiveness, and allowing the next stage of our relationship to blossom.

I'm lost. In limbo. I feel this anger, frustration, and heartache will consume me. I no longer feel that I am doing Jessica any good as I sit by her. I am no longer able to concentrate on the Light. I don't make it to the end of the week before I'm running to my car in tears, heading north, seeking a cave deep in the wilderness in which I can hide, scream, cry, and sleep.

Halfway to Oregon, I sit on the coast of California, watching the waves crash into the shore. I breathe in the pure air and hope, wish, and pray the angry sea will carry away my heartache.

I won't stay away long. Though my own abandonment issues run to my core, I can never let my daughters down like that.

I will go back to my difficult and tragic life, but somehow, please, at the end of this disaster, let me find peace.

VARIATION DEUX

Love me when I least deserve it, because that's when I need it the most.

Swedish Proverb

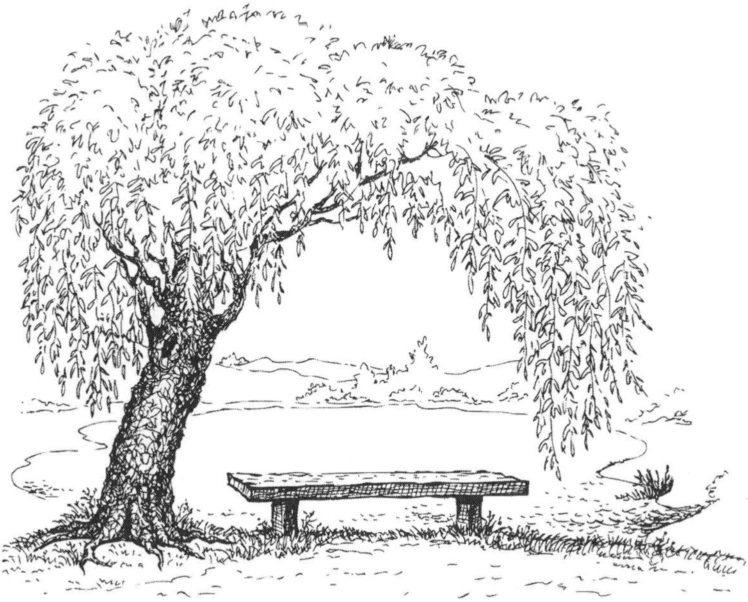

CHAPTER TWENTY-EIGHT

The Hourglass on the Table

The caller ID shows a 734 prefix again, so I eagerly answer, knowing it's someone in the UC Davis Health System.

"May I speak to the parent or guardian of Jessica Lavine?"

"That's me."

"Hello, Ms. Lavine, this is Libby from Dr Lee's office. We're ready to schedule Jessica's bone flap replacement."

"Oh! Yes! Thank you!" I jump out of my seat and grab the marker for the whiteboard.

"Jessica is scheduled for surgery this Wednesday, October 27, 2010. You will receive a phone call Tuesday night to confirm the time and review the pre-op instructions. You will also need to take Jessica to the lab at the Lawrence J. Ellison Ambulatory Care Center any time on Tuesday to have pre-op labs drawn."

I scribble this information on the white board, conclude the call, and immediately phone Jesse to share the good news.

"Wouldn't it be great if they took her straight from the bone-flap replacement to inpatient rehab?" I ask. The four of us are sitting in the waiting room on the morning of Jessica's long-awaited operation.

"Yeah, but I doubt that will happen. Manhart said it would be another three months after this procedure."

"Oh, yeah. She'll need to recover and regain her stamina."

"Well, at least we can look forward to it being sooner rather than later."

"Jessica Lavine?" A nurse shows up at the door of the waiting room, and we collect our things.

"I'll take Jocelyn to the cafeteria while you get her settled in," Jesse tells me.

"Sounds good, I'll meet you there."

"Ms. Lavine?" A tall woman with a Dutch accent pulls open the curtain to Jessica's pre-op area. Decked out in scrubs and holding a clipboard, she reaches out to shake my hand. "It's good to see you again."

"Good morning, Dr. Lee."

"Good morning. So we're ready to get Jessica all fixed up?"

"Yes, finally." I smile at her.

"Great. We're about ready to get started. The entire process should take about an hour and a half, and then she will go to recovery. You will be able to sit with her while she wakes up."

"Okay, great. Thank you."

She drifts away, meeting up with the nurses on her way through the doors I assume lead to the operating suites.

I sit down and adjust the hospital cap the nurses have placed on Thomy's head to help put Jessica at ease. I grab Jessica's hand and sing quietly to her.

"You are my sunshine, my only sunshine..."

"Are you sure she said an hour and a half?" Jesse asks at the three-hour mark.

We've had breakfast in the café, and he's dropped Jocelyn off at daycare. We've taken a walk outside, checked email and Facebook on our phones, flipped through magazines, and wrung our hands dry.

"She did. Should we check in? Maybe she's already in recovery, and we missed them coming to get us."

"I don't see how we would have. I'll ask." He heads over to the check-in desk to speak with the clerk. I chew on my lip and adjust our bags again.

"She says she's not in recovery yet."

"It's taken twice as long as Dr. Lee said. I hope everything is going okay."

Jesse pulls his chair closer and puts his arm around me. "I'm sure it's fine."

I lean on his shoulder and attempt to take a nap while time creeps by.

After five and a half hours, Dr. Lee emerges from the door where they took Jessica into pre-op. "Hello, Mr. and Ms. Lavine. I apologize for the lengthy time."

I sit forward, eager to learn how my girl is doing. "Is everything okay?"

"Yes, Jessica is doing great. She did very well." Dr. Lee sits down in the chair near us and leans in close. "The reason surgery took so long is due to the amount of time it has been since Jessica's accident. Her skull had begun to regenerate. When I went to put in the prosthetic, it did not fit."

"Is that common?" Jesse asked. "Should we have known?"

"It happens, but not very often. Jessica had about a half inch of growth."

"Half an inch! Wow." I'm stunned by my daughter's ability to heal her body. "So what did you do? Were you able to fix her head?"

"Yes. It took about three hours for me to grind the prosthetic down and refit it to the new space. Once we had that done, everything else went as planned. She is in recovery now. Would you like to be with her?"

"Yes, please." We stand and follow her.

Though Dr. Lee told us in our pre-op meeting that she would only need to shave the part of Jessica's skull where they were performing the operation, something else must have changed. Jessica's head is clearly clean-shaven under the bandages that cover her head.

"Oh, sweet girl," I whisper. Sitting next to the bed, I sing to her again, relieved that her beautiful brain is protected and she is whole once again.

"Hey, guys. How's it going?"

"Hey! Jessica, Faye is here to see you."

As soon as Jessica woke up, they transported us from the surgical wing up to the pediatric floor. A small smile emerges on Jessica's face, and her eyes open a little more.

"She still out of it a bit?"

"Yeah. They said the operation went well, though. Now we can move on to getting her into inpatient therapy."

"Did they tell you when that would happen?"

I shrug and sit in the ever-present chair-bed.

"Manhart said probably three months after her head is fixed. I was kind of hoping to get her straight in . . ." I gesture toward Jess's swollen face and head. "But I see now that I wasn't thinking it through. She'll obviously need to recover first."

"Also, we're coming up on the holidays, so the scheduling gets wonky," Faye says. "Maybe they'll move it up to January, but I really don't see it happening before then."

"Yeah." I sigh. "Soon, I guess, though."

"Before you know it. Well, I gotta get going."

I stand to give her a hug. "Thanks for coming by to see her. We'll see you again soon."

"Sure thing!" she calls over her shoulder on her way out the door.

"Hello?" an accented voice calls. I wake to footsteps coming into the room. "Is this..."

It's Joan, the neurosurgery nurse practitioner who saved Jessica's life the day after the accident. I jump to my feet to greet her. "Hi. Yes, this is Jessica. Do you remember her?"

Joan shoves her notes into the pocket of her lab coat and brings a hand to her mouth. "Of course,... I'm so sorry." She turns toward the window, and I move to stand next to her, a lump in my throat.

"Don't be sorry." When I put my hand on her shoulder, she turns to me, and we hug one another tight.

"I'm so sorry. I shouldn't be..." Her voice is muffled by her tears.

"Don't worry about it. I'm so glad to have the chance to thank you. Thank you for saving her life. Thank you." I squeeze her tight and then release her.

She wipes her eyes and moves to the bed to examine Jessica.

"Hello, Jessica. Your mom and I were just having a moment. How are you doing?" Her professionalism returns, and she retrieves her notes and begins the examination while repeating her question to me. "How is she doing?"

"Pretty good. Just groggy and in a little pain from the operation. Overall, she's doing really well." I tell her a little bit about the progress Jessica is making and the therapy she's been getting at home and at an outpatient facility in Folsom.

"Squeeze my hand, Jessica. As hard as you can." Then she asks me, "And you're happy with the therapy? You don't want to do inpatient therapy? What are your goals for her?"

I can't correct her quickly enough. "Oh, no, no. We *do* want to do inpatient therapy. Dr. Manhart said the timing would depend on how soon she recovers."

"Mm-hmmm." She does more of the routine tests all the doctors and therapists put Jessica through: tracking her finger, squeezing her hands, lifting and moving her arms and legs. "Well, she is obviously strong enough and ready for inpatient, so you want to wait?"

"What? No! Not at all."

"Okay. I'll be right back." She makes some notes on her paper and strides out of the room, determination in her step.

I stand there, momentarily stunned, and then pick up my phone and text Jesse.

Um, we just had a visit from Joan the neurosurgery NP. I think if she has her way, we won't see the light of day for a few weeks.

What? Why's that?

I think she's getting us admitted for inpatient.

Omg!

"What are you doing?" Faye has returned, this time carrying her backpack and the ever-present page of notes.

"Are we staying?"

"I'm here to do an evaluation, so I guess you're staying."

"Holy crap, that was fast."

"I know; what happened?"

"Joan from neurosurgery came and examined Jess. I knew we were going to get in. She looked determined when she left."

"Well, congrats. I never thought it would happen this way."

"Me either. We came in expecting to stay one or two nights, not one or two weeks."

"It may be even longer than that. You remember how things can change."

"Obviously minute to minute."

I relax in the chair-bed and let her do her evaluation. Staying for rehab right after such a major surgery does seem a little soon, but we've been wanting this for so long. I can't help but be excited for this next chapter in Jessica's recovery.

CHAPTER TWENTY-NINE

Make Me Lighter

I'm aching for tools that are strictly prohibited in the hospital: some sage to burn, a few candles to light, or even a stick of incense to set ablaze on the small bedside table.

I know it doesn't matter that I don't physically have my desired sacred objects here. Harnessing the light and energy that has been sent to us since Jessica's accident has been just as easy without something tangible in my hands. That doesn't keep me from wishing I could add a little more balance to the sterile air in this cold room.

Once we learned we would be admitted for inpatient therapy, I asked Jesse to bring some items from home. I set about arranging the items, which includes pictures of Jessica, my Angels, Willow Tree figurines, gifts from visitors, and a few items that have been with us since Jessica's birth. Gathered together, they create a little altar in her room.

Little altars everywhere.

I try to keep this practice going, bringing a small sense of grace and reverence to any room we occupy; I fill the spaces to make it feel like home.

As overjoyed as we were to have Jessica admitted for inpatient therapy, our second round of hospital life has been a bit of a wake-up call. I've come to terms with the fact that much of the wait-and-see we have been dealing with since her accident is over.

We were waiting for her head to be fixed, waiting for her to start following commands, waiting for her to respond to yes/no questions, waiting for inpatient rehab…all leading up to waiting for her to be better.

Now her head is fixed.

She follows commands when she feels like it. She is fully capable but doesn't always listen.

She has yes/no communication and is beginning to communicate with some sign language and Augmentative and Alternative Communication (AAC) devices.

Wait-and-see continues, and I'm shutting down. I struggle to find the words to keep people updated. I feel I have no strength, energy, spirit, or even fight left in me. I know these qualities are essential to moving through this process, but hospital life is draining.

The progress Jessica is making in inpatient rehab isn't as rapid as we dreamed it would be, which is disheartening.

Life is settling into something quiet and isolated, making it necessary to dig deep to find the resources to keep going day to day.

"Knock knock." Barb comes through the door of Jessica's hospital room carrying a shopping bag. "Where's Jessica?"

"Hey." I get up from my chair-bed to greet her with a hug. "In therapy. I stayed back today. I needed some time alone."

"Are you okay? I brought you lunch."

"Thank you. I didn't feel like heading down to the cafeteria." We sit at the round table on the side of Jessica's bed opposite my chair-bed, and Barb pulls soup and salad from the bag.

"So how is it going?"

"Okay." I nod to confirm my response as I take a bite and then sit back.

"Just okay?"

I nod again and swallow. "No, not just okay. Jessica's doing really well. She's making good progress in here. It's just…" I shrug and take another bite.

"Now's when the hard work begins?" Barb suggests.

"Yes," I agree through a mouthful of salad. Covering my mouth with my hand, I stifle a laugh. "Sorry. But yes. That's pretty much the perfect way to describe it. I'm so proud of all the progress she's made, but boy do we have so far to go."

"You know she'll get there."

"I know she will."

We continue our lunch, sharing memories of Bench Time at dance, and she tells me news about her children, Hannah and Max. As we finish our meal, she pulls a stack of papers from the shopping bag.

"So, I did want to talk to you about the fundraiser I told you about at recital."

Perplexed by the pile of papers, I raise my eyebrows. "I thought we were going to do a bake sale or a car wash or something."

She laughs at me and scoots her chair closer so we can go through the papers together. "Yeah, no. Here's what we have."

I am astonished at the event Barb has pulled together. A pasta feed at the community center in Folsom. She has been selling tickets for an all-you-can-eat pasta, bread, salad, and dessert event and shows me the list of donations for a silent auction. "There will also be a no-host bar with water, soda, beer, and wine, and we'll sell raffle tickets throughout the night."

I read the list of donations, which includes big-ticket items like a three-night stay at a cabin in Lake Tahoe, a mystery case of wine provided by regulars on the MyFolsom forum I've posted on for seven years, a dance workshop with Ms. Melissa, and much more. "Barb, I don't know what to say."

"You have done so much for so many people over the years; it's time to let the community help you."

My heart catches in my throat, and I feel my fog lift a bit.

CHAPTER THIRTY

Jumpstart My Kaleidoscope Heart

"Jolene?" A man with salt-and-pepper hair steps into the waiting room of the office building where I'm sitting. Jesse took over for me at the hospital so I could make it to my own therapy appointment.

"Yes." I stand up and reach out to shake his hand. "David?"

"Yes. Come on back."

"Thanks." I follow him down the hall and into a small office. "Where should I sit?"

"Wherever you like."

I take a seat on the brown leather couch. As he gets settled across from me, I admire the artwork on the wall behind him.

"So, how can I help you?" he begins.

I meet his eyes and laugh. "Oh, Lord. I'm not sure."

I do the best I can to give him a concise history of Jessica's accident, the progress she's made so far, being back in inpatient therapy, and how I've been feeling lately.

"How *are* you feeling lately?"

"Honestly? I don't know. Part of me doesn't care. I feel kind of numb."

"What are you angry about?"

"I didn't say angry. I said numb." I'm aware of the edge in my voice.

"Can I tell you what I call being numb?" He doesn't wait for me to take a guess but presses on. "Anger in denial."

I start to zone out as he reviews concepts I'm familiar with.

Therapy stuff I've understood for some time but haven't had much success integrating into my life lately.

I sigh and apologize. "I'm sorry. I realize I'm a difficult patient. Even though I'm willing to look at my behavior, change what needs to be changed, learn new ways of tackling problems, and accept when something hasn't been working for me, I'm also argumentative and unsure of my own abilities. I have a fear of success and have unlocked the master level of self-sabotage."

David shifts in his seat, gives me an obligatory chuckle, and asks bluntly, "Where has that gotten you in the past? Where do you want to be? Will that self-sabotage get you there?"

"Well. No."

"Right. Good answer. Our time is almost up, but let me tell you I'd like to help you. However, I can only help you if you're ready. You can spend a lot of time tiptoeing around what you need to do and talking about being committed to change. Until you decide that you are committed, you'll stay stuck. So think about that, and then call me to set up your next appointment when you decide you are ready to move forward."

While I consider the option he's laid out for me, I stare at him, trying to determine: *friend or foe*? "Okay. I'll give you a call."

We handle payment for the session, and I gather my purse and head out of the office. I text Jesse to tell him I'm on my way back to the hospital, unlock the car, get in, and turn the key.

Sara Bareilles' voice greets me with confirmation of the message David shared with me, and I pull out of the parking lot and head for the freeway.

Compare where you are to where you want to be, and you'll get nowhere.

CHAPTER THIRTY-ONE

Be You in Time

I'm barely through the door of Jessica's room before Jesse is greeting me. "Okay, I know you are tired of hospital life, and this inpatient stay hasn't been as miraculous as you would have liked, but I have some good news for you."

"Oh?" I set my purse down and kiss Jessica's face. She is already laughing and doing her bed dance, shaking her body all around.

"She took her first steps!"

"What!" I mentally kick myself for daring to leave the hospital. "Tell me! No, wait. Write this down!" I sit at the round table where Barb and I ate lunch and shove my laptop at him.

"You never get to see things like this. I'm so glad it happened for you. Write it down to go on the Facebook page."

"Okay." He settles into the chair, and I read over his shoulder while he types.

During Jessica's physical therapy session, her therapists had Jessica attempt to use the parallel bars for the first time. They are a set of bars about thirty feet long.

They wheeled her to one end and had her grip the bars with her hands. Her right hand, actually, since she is still working on full control of the left one. With maximum support, they helped her into a standing position.

"Maximum" support is just want it sounds like. Although Jessica was bearing most of the weight on her own two feet, one therapist stood in front of her, holding her hips straight, while another one stood behind her, holding her shoulders back.

And then—she just about fell down. Before anyone was ready, she threw her right leg forward, and the therapist in front of her had to catch her. They got her steadied and then, slowly, had her take a step forward with her right foot. Then they had to bring her left foot forward for her, as she is still working on control of that side. Then she took her second step forward on her own.

After that, they took a break. Throughout it all, she was having quite a bit of discomfort; some of those muscles haven't been used in months, so she obviously needed a rest. We asked her if it hurt, and she nodded yes. We asked her if she wanted to try again, and she nodded an emphatic yes.

She ended up taking four more steps forward on her own, or about half the length of the bars.

He hits Publish and turns to grin at me. I look at Jessica, who is laughing and wiggling in the bed again. "Oh, Jess! I'm so proud of you! Was that awesome?"

She nods at me, and the delight is evident in her eyes. I grin from ear to ear and pull the laptop back from Jesse to watch the likes and comments come spilling in.

"I should probably give them updates on some of the other stuff that's happened."

"You should," Jesse agrees.

Jessica has been wearing splints on her hands at night to help keep them flat so that she doesn't develop contractures. One morning, as I was in the bathroom getting ready for our day, I heard the sound of Velcro ripping and stepped out into the room to see Jessica with the strap from one of the splints in her mouth. Faye called it problem solving.

Along the same lines, in her physical therapy session with Señor Jack, he held his hand about six inches above her leg and asked her to bring her leg to his hand. Instead, Jessica put her right hand on Jack's and pushed it to her leg. Problem solving again!

In a combination of occupational therapy and physical therapy, they have been putting Jessica in a contraption called a LiteGait. A harness supports Jessica's torso, and there are handles for her to hold onto. When the therapists roll the LiteGait forward, it forces Jessica to bear weight on and move her legs. The LiteGait will also help improve her neck muscles so she can gain better head control. This will speed her recovery in many areas: sitting, standing, walking, and eating.

Jessica screamed during the entire first time in the LiteGait, but after seven weeks, she is all smiles and eager to work every time they roll it out.

The biggest improvement, however, is in Jessica's swallowing. While the speech therapist, Michelle, has been working with Jessica on different AAC devices, the other speech therapists, Kim and Ann, have been working on Jessica's swallow reflex. They have fed her yogurt, pudding, ice cream, thickened liquids, and graham crackers soaked in milk, all with good results.

They also performed a swallow study in which Jessica ate foods and drank liquids containing barium while they used an x-ray to determine how she is swallowing. The results were such that Jessica has graduated to a diet of thickened liquids and soft/pureed foods.

Will 7:00 be too late to come for a visit?

Absolutely not! Please! We miss you and Hannah.

GREAT! Is there anything I can bring the baby girl? Since she can eat food now? How about a Frosty from Wendy's?

Great idea! She will love that! See you later! I love you. XO

See you soon. XOXOXOXO

"Hi, honey! How are things going?" Kari and Hannah arrive with the promised Wendy's dinner and treats. I hug Kari tight and kiss Hannah on the top of the head.

"Better," I admit, taking the bag she gives me, which contains a salad and a soda. "Thank you."

"Oh, I'm glad. Do you want me to do this while you eat?" She holds up the Frosty meant for Jessica.

"Oh, I don't know. I don't think Jessica remembers chocolate Frosties from Wendy's. I don't think she'll want it." To prove my claims wrong, Jessica starts laughing and yelling and dancing in the bed again.

"Get it, girl!" Kari tells her and starts dancing for Jessica.

"Uh-oh, Jess! Look what you started. Auntie's going to bust a move up in here."

"Maybe after her Frosty," Kari says as she raises the head of Jessica's bed. "So things are going better?" she asks again as she feeds Jessica a small spoonful.

"Yeah." I bring her up to date on the progress Jesse and I have been posting about on Facebook.

"I read! I'm so proud of you, Jess! Trying to get walking already."

"Yeah. Jesse is right. As inconvenient and difficult as the hospital stay has been this time around, I'm glad we're here. These therapists are pushing Jessica hard and not letting her get out of things easily. It is paying off. Her strength is increasing daily, and the therapists are eager to try bigger and better things with her every day."

"That's great. And she's working hard?"

"For the most part." I start grinning.

"What?" She knows me too well.

"There have been some roadblocks here and there. Jessica has gotten comfortable with the therapists, so she is relearning how to assert her independence and is fighting them half the time. As much as I want to tell her to get it together, it is nice because it reminds me of how she was before the accident."

"Oh, yes. She could be very headstrong, that's for sure. She wants to do things her own way."

"Yep. Today, Faye had Jessica lying on her back on the mat. Then she put a beanbag in Jessica's hand and instructed her to reach above her head and put the bean bag in a bucket that was at the top of the mat."

"To work on her range of motion."

"Right. You know that, being a therapist and all. Anyway, Jess did pretty well at first, but as she got more tired, it was more difficult for her."

"Of course."

"But you know her. She didn't want to stop until she had put all of those beanbags in that bucket."

"I can just see it!" Kari giggles.

"It reminded me of one time in dance class when the girls were working on their double leaps. Melissa made them do those leaps over and over again, and Jessica got mad. She was so tired, and she stood there in line at the barre, waiting her turn with her hands on her hips and blowing air in a huff.

"Melissa asked her if she needed a break, and she straight up told her, 'No, I will get this. I just need to get mad enough.' I feel like if she could talk now, she would have said the same thing to Faye today."

Kari gives Jessica her attention again and half lectures her. "Girl, you need to listen to your therapists. They are working hard to help you get better. It will help more if you cooperate."

Jessica giggles in response and says, "Uh-huh."

Kari and I look at each other.

"What? Did she just say what I think she said?"

"Uh-huh," She says again.

I jump up from my seat. "Oh, my goodness!"

"Go, Jessica! It's your birthday!" Kari starts chanting and doing a little dance. I grab her hips to form a Conga line, and Hannah brings up the rear. We dance around the room, singing, "Uh-huh, raise the roof. Uh-huh, shake your groove thing. Uh-huh, get your groove on, uh-huh!"

Jessica dances in the bed and laughs so hard she starts coughing.

"Oh, no! Are you okay?" I turn on the suction machine and hold the suction tube at the ready.

Jessica coughs a little more, and then says, "Uh-huh."

We all start laughing again.

A visit with our girls is precisely what the doctor ordered. Having Kari help with Jessica's care and seeing Hannah treat her with sweet cousinly love. Watching them be goofy together, giggling and even just lying together in Jessica's bed, their heads close together, looking into one another's eyes.

As I settle into bed that evening, I text Kari again:

Thank you for the therapy session. Your love helps Jessica gain so much strength. I cannot thank you enough.

Of course. We love you all. Oh, check in your purse. Barb gave me something to drop off to you. Sleep well tonight. We'll see you soon. XOXO XOXOXO

I put the phone down and grab my purse from the floor. I fish out the envelope Kari must be talking about and open it up. Inside is a check and a note from Barb.

It was a great night. The big winners were the Walker family. They won the auctions on the cabin in Tahoe, as well as a beach house at Sea Ranch and a B&B in Sacramento. Jessica's cousins, dance friends, and Girl Scout troop did a great job serving. The Folsom Mounted Police and the Grace Foundation have donated six months of therapeutic riding lessons for Jessica. 250 people. Your girl is well loved.

I set the letter aside and unfold the check. I have to cover my mouth to stifle the gasp so I don't wake Jessica. I grab my phone and quietly head out to the hall so I can call Jesse.

He picks up on the first ring. "Hi, honey."

"Hey, so, um. Can you please go by Best Buy tomorrow and pick up the iPad for Jessica like we've been talking about?"

"Can we afford that?" He sounds bewildered.

"Yes. I got a check from Barb for the pasta feed today."

"Oh? And?"

"$15,000.00."

"Holy shit."

"I know!"

"Okay, yeah. I'll see you guys tomorrow with the iPad."

It's my turn to update the Viva La Jessica! page on Facebook again.

Dearest family and friends,

Thank you for attending the pasta feed this weekend. Jesse and I are blown away by your generosity.

The money raised at the pasta feed will help pay our out-of-pocket portion for a properly fitting wheelchair for Jessica; foot orthotics, which will help keep her feet in the proper position so when the time comes to stand and walk again, she can do so with greater ease; therapies once our insurance cuts off, as we have been warned it will; and, most importantly, an iPad and the ProLoQ app that will help with Jessica's rapidly increasing awareness and her ability to communicate.

Since Jessica's accident, we have been attempting to express our gratitude for everything that has been done for our family. We may have to accept the fact this is an impossible feat.

It will not stop us from trying.

Thank you to everyone who has been there for us throughout this life-changing tragedy. We believe in the power of love, positive thought and prayer. As such, we would not be where we are without you. Thank you for your support of our girl and for lifting her up to the Light for Healing. We greatly appreciate each of you.

Love,

The Lavine Family

CHAPTER THIRTY-TWO

Closer Than You Think

"Can I ask again?" David begins gently.

I've made the call, and I'm back on the leather couch in his office. I thought about what he said in our first meeting and ultimately decided he is right.

Regardless of circumstance, intent, and whatever else is going on in my head, heart, and life, if I am committed to making things better for myself, my husband, and our daughters, then I need to make some changes.

My current habits do not serve me well. My moods, my weight, my fitness level, and the commitment to all aspects of my life are not acceptable. Something needs to change.

I can't be committed in my head and then drink a six-pack, eat a pint of Ben & Jerry's, screw around on the computer for hours, and wonder why things aren't changing. Taking the time to make small changes day by day may not be perfect, but at least I can feel committed to change.

"Ask what?" I ask him once I've gotten up the nerve.

"What are you angry about?"

I feel the urge to resume the numb-versus-angry argument with him but keep myself in check. Instead, I take a moment to think about the question. "I'm going to actually try here. Give me a sec, okay?"

"Of course; take your time."

Closing my eyes, I imagine all that has happened since Jessica's accident and all I want to have happen. All that truly matters to me is Jessica and how she will recover, her therapy, and what we need and want to do. *So what am I angry about?*

My hands instinctively find the Om mudra, and in my mind's eye I see the long-lost threads of energy flowing from Mother Earth and The Universe, nudging my stubborn chakras. *What am I always so angry about?*

"Stupid, dramatic bullshit, really." These words, simple and blunt, sum up the distractions in my life.

"How so?" He presses.

"I keep getting caught up in these interactions that honestly, obviously make a difference in my life, since I have emotional energy to expend on them, but..."

"Like what? What interactions?"

I shift in my seat, hands on my lap and palms up, searching for the appropriate example. "Just a few weeks ago, I was telling my husband about a lady who accused me of the most random stuff. Like being mad at her about good things going on in her life. I engaged in an argument with her for a few minutes before just stepping away and realizing it didn't really matter. Later, I recognized it as a good distraction from the bigger stuff going on in my life, but, honestly, the argument itself didn't matter."

"Is that the only one? The only..." He checks his notepad to get the wording right. "'...stupid, dramatic bullshit'?"

"Not the only one, but, really, they're all the same. Interactions with people who don't really think about what they're saying before they say it. The specifics don't matter. It's the emotions of the interactions that break my heart and make me resentful."

"Resentful of what?"

I look at him, press my lips together, and just shake my head. We watch each other for a minute before he takes a drink of water, shifts his position, and tries again. "These interactions... they are with different people? Or the same person?"

"A few different people."

"And despite what happened, you're resentful because...?"

I bite my lip, shake my head, and look up at the ceiling, willing my eyes not to fill with tears. David leans forward and gently pushes the box of Kleenex on the bookshelf toward me. I snatch a couple out of the box.

"Well, now I'm mad because I'm upset. I don't have time to deal with this. That's why it's easier to just go numb."

"Again, how's that working out for you?"

More head shaking as I dab at the corners of my eyes and sniffle quietly.

"I get resentful..." I start slowly, trying to keep my voice even. "...over the fact that because of Jessica's accident...I feel like we've paid up everything."

"What do you mean?"

"I thought..." My voice breaks, and the tears start falling. "... my heartache was transparent. I wear my emotions on my sleeve. Can't the world see me walking around, bleeding, sobbing, aching, and desperate desperate *desperate* for a touch? A hug? Some help. A savior. Someone to hold me and let me cry until I can't cry anymore?"

I pause to blow my nose and wipe my face. "Can't they see that and not tell me, in the most devastating of ways, how horrible a person I am and that they don't have time for a relationship with me, because it's never going to work?

"Or just drop our friendship for reasons I can only imagine but am never told?

"I didn't expect the people I thought knew me best to assume the worst about my behavior and cut me off at the knees without even taking the chance to hear what could have possibly been going on with me. Doesn't everyone see? Isn't it obvious?"

"What's obvious?" David asks gently.

"I swing in a limbo of perpetual grief. No closure from death, no joy at a complete recovery. Simply living with the constant reminder of what we once had, struggling to accept what will be.

"I long for normal, the old, the familiar. For Bench Time or ritual, beers in the hot tub, or even a hug after the death of a loved one."

"A kind word."

I nod furiously at him, wiping my dripping nose again.

"But no. The loss of our life before is apparently not enough, and the blows continue to come. Judgment for how I'm handling this horrific situation, reminders of past transgressions, condemnation for daring to feel the magnitude of the feelings that course through me on a daily basis."

"It's a lot," he comments.

More nodding.

"The misunderstandings occur, and the abyss grows. People continue to disappear, and I retreat further into my cave. I wish away this hole in my chest, the void where the hurricane swept through and wiped away *everything* I was so in love with. Everything I was grateful for. The brilliant lights in my life snuffed out in a heartbeat.

"I try to hold onto all of the good, the communities of people who have given their time, heart, and soul to us and the Love and Light being slung toward our family constantly. I hope and pray and work to manifest my own love, strength, and healing. Sometimes, sometimes I think it would be easier to let go if I were able to call people out on their bullshit and petty behavior, but they can't understand, so it's easier to Just. Go. Numb."

"But that's not working," David reminds me gently. Then he asks, "What don't they understand?"

"Our life. They don't have to live this. I'm living this. Jesse is living this. They don't have to. No one else has to get up at 5:00 a.m. to prepare medications and 'breakfast,' which consists of a milky white formula traveling through a tube straight into my daughter's stomach.

"Sponge baths. Physical therapy in bed. Wishing for more and more assistance, hoping someone can come and wave a magic wand, to be a catalyst for our Hollywood moment. To create another miracle.

"To make my daughter dance again." I close my eyes, hoping

to block out the memories of recitals, performances, competitions, rehearsals. "We're living this. They're not. They are dealing with their own demons. Their own sicknesses, deaths, financial troubles, and traumatic events..."

"You don't think they can imagine how hard it is on you?" David's look is gentle, whether carefully crafted after years on the job or truly feeling for me doesn't matter. He is clearly trying to understand. That makes all the difference.

"I don't think they can. Jessica lived. Doesn't that make everything perfect?" I take a moment to breathe. I look at the tissues in my hand and fold them over and over again, making them as small as I can before opening them back up and repeating the process. "It's funny. I have had friends tell me how much they appreciate how authentic, honest, and real I am."

"That seems nice to me, not funny."

"Well, yeah." A small smile. Fold. Fold. Fold. "The funny part is what I've learned over the years, through all of these petty interactions. No one really wants this. They don't want this *real*," I state, complete with air quotes. "A grief so heavy you can't move. The sound of the tearing of your soul is deafening. The quality and quantity of your tears are overwhelming in their frequency and duration."

He stares while I shred my tissues.

"No one wants this real. Certainly no one knows how to handle it. It is the most isolating part of this process. We have the love and support of so many people, yet the care and understanding my heart and soul need are elusive.

"Our lives changed so dramatically, and we have lost so much. We've gained a lot, yes, but major, major parts of our lives, including people who have been there for us for years, have changed."

"You're changing, too." Such a simple and obvious response.

"Yeah." I listen to the clock tick.

I am. I have.

My breath steadies, and I set the tissues on the couch next to me. I feel the familiar, gentle nudge of the Angelic beings, and my voice softens. "I'm angry that people haven't seen my changes. I'm not who I've always been."

"How could you be?"

Shrug. Breathe. Nudge.

"I feel so broken…"

Eyes closed. Heart beating. Resting in the soft support of Divine Intervention.

David's voice finds me through the mist. "Maybe the pieces needed to break away…"

"So the Me I'm meant to be could be free," I whisper.

Nudge.

Nod.

Breathe.

CHAPTER THIRTY-THREE

I Will Lay Me Down

I sit close to Jessica's bed, configuring her new iPad and showing her how to use the speech app we downloaded for her.

She reaches out to push some of the icons I've created for her and laughs at the robotic voice coming from the speaker.

My name is Jessica.

I am ten years old.

My favorite color is purple.

"If you push this button, you can type in whatever you want." I push the keyboard icon and type in a sentence. "Then touch the Speak button."

Hello, Jessica, this is Mom.

She giggles and pulls the iPad closer to her lap to begin playing with it independently. I fiddle with my phone while she explores. A few minutes pass, and I hear Jessica giggling.

"What's up?" I lean forward to see what mischief she's getting into.

Sutcase.

"Do you mean suitcase?" I ask her, and she giggles and nods. "Okay. Remember, it's spelled s-u-i-t-c-a-s-e." I spell for her while typing it out on the iPad.

"Now what about it?"

She motions toward the closet with her eyes.

"Right, that's where the suitcase is. What about it?"

She looks at the closet again, and I raise my eyebrows and look at the iPad. She huffs and touches the screen.

Pack. Home.

I can't help but smile from ear to ear. We have communication.

"I'm proud of you, but we're not going home yet. Do you want to take the suitcase to therapy tomorrow?"

She nods and looks quite pleased with herself.

On Friday nights, Jesse leaves work early so I have a chance to get a break from hospital life. He and Jocelyn entertain Jessica while I go home and spend some time alone and sleep in a real bed before returning to the hospital in the morning.

When he and Jocelyn arrive, Jessica is excited to see him and signs *Dad* over and over again before pushing all of the buttons on the iPad for him.

He and Jocelyn join Jessica on the bed while I pack up the overnight bag with my computer and the dirty clothes I will take home and trade out for clean ones. I sit and watch the three of them for a minute.

I'm grateful for the strength and support Jesse lends me. As excited as I am for Jessica and the progress she is making, it is getting increasingly difficult for me to remain positive when I'm sitting here with her every day. Most days it feels impossibly hard.

People keep telling me how strong and brave I am, but they wouldn't say that if they were here with me. I sense myself losing it more and more every day. I wake up confident in a new day and the possibilities ahead. Changes, new advances, the progress she makes for the therapist . . . anything. It's a brand new day.

By noon, I'm dead tired and beaten down and ready for a break. On days like today, I look forward to a small break, which I hope will eliminate even a sliver of the stress of our lives. I kiss my family on their heads and leave the room.

I'm also grateful for the nights like tonight, when Jesse and I hit the sweet spot that has only come around every couple of months since Jessica's accident. We're going on five years of marriage, and I feel so blessed to know if our circumstances were different, we'd still be running around like teenagers in love. It is the strength of our connection that is holding our family together through this nightmare.

That connection has always been perfect when we make love, but these days I often find sex to be therapeutic, as well. When we get the chance to connect, touch, and talk, I feel safe enough to relax more than I'm able to do at any other point in our chaotically busy lives. I wish the logistics worked out for it to happen more often.

After a day full of work for Jesse, therapy and doctors' appointments for Jessica and me, and trying to squeeze some sort of normal into our lives for Jocelyn, our evening routine ends with Jesse going to bed early enough to get up for work. I stay up, watching episode after episode of *The Office* or *Grey's Anatomy* on Netflix and playing any of the dozens of "Dash" games to occupy my mind.

Television and games aren't a complete fix for the overwhelming depression and grief that still plague me day to day, but they allow me to zone out until exhaustion takes over and I'm able to stumble to bed and fall asleep immediately, rather than lying there choking on *whys*, wishing for a little *because*.

With the passing of each week, I try to keep the faith that our daily life will eventually allow Jesse and me to do more than barely touch one another before giving into the never-ending fatigue the end of the day brings.

Entering the dark house, I set the overnight bag next to the hallway and go to the kitchen to heat some water for tea. I walk from room to room, formulating a plan of attack on the housework that isn't sympathetic to our daily plight. I only have a couple of hours, so I won't be able to do the deep cleaning the house desperately needs. I'm happy to be able to catch up on laundry, clean up the kitchen, and even throw together some freezer meals for the coming week.

Feeling accomplished and grateful to be able to contribute to the upkeep of the household, I jump in a hot shower, hoping in vain to rinse away the parts of my day that cling to me like a second skin. Feeling red and raw, with my soul wrung out, I climb into bed and open up the Netflix app on my phone.

When Jesse finally gets home, he enters so quietly that I assume Jocelyn must have fallen asleep on the way home. Sure enough, he comes to our room moments later, changes his clothes, and slips into bed.

"Hi, baby." He snuggles up close to me and nuzzles his face into my hair.

I pause my show and turn to kiss him, grateful to no longer be alone. "How was Jess's evening? Who's her nurse tonight?"

"Jessica Y. is her night nurse. Our Jess is doing fine. I helped get her changed and ready for sleep before leaving."

"You didn't wait for her to fall asleep?"

"It's impossible for her while Jocelyn is still there."

I nod in the dark and turn my attention to my phone, setting the alarm in the hope of getting up early enough to reach the hospital before Jessica wakes. I hate the thought of her waking up without Jesse or me there to greet the day with her.

"Well, I'm going to try to read a little bit," he says, "but I'm pretty tired."

"I know."

I turn to him and touch his face, running my fingers along his bearded jawline. "Thank you for relieving me at the hospital tonight. I realize driving out there after you've worked all day is a lot to ask—"

"Don't." He pushes my hair away from my face and pulls me closer. "You're at the hospital with Jessica every day. I wish I could come out more often."

I shake my head and allow his strength to hold me together. I can't fathom the thought of him feeling like he needs to do more. He works full time, shuttles Jocelyn to daycare each day, and brings me clothes and meals at the hospital every other day, never seeming to break his stride.

"You already do so much," I whisper into his chest, enjoying the movement of his fingers in my hair.

"You're my family; what else would I do?"

I'm not sure what else to say and probably shouldn't try to argue with him anyway. I reach behind me to put the phone on my nightstand, giving into the relaxation of his light massage on my neck. He pulls me close, and within seconds our breathing is in sync. Within minutes, we are moving together.

The hungry hands that grip our days are like a vice, squeezing out any chance for peace or joy. In these precious moments we're able to steal away, it doesn't take long for us to find a comfort and safety in the warmth of each other's hearts.

Usually the release of our intimacy is welcome, and the type of exhaustion it brings allows me to fall asleep in a euphoric state rather than the usual drastic fatigue. It is a cruel world, however, when that works against me.

I sigh as we kiss, relax as Jesse touches me, and by the end of it all, my defenses are weakened. The shell I've created around the pain of losing the life we had starts to crack. The wall I've constructed to keep the grief of losing Pre-Accident Jessica from overwhelming me starts to crumble. By the time we reach our stormy haze, I realize how weakened I am. Instead of floating off to sleep, I am overwhelmed by sobs.

This isn't anything new.

The release of stress and tension that comes from being so close is definitely welcome. There are instances like this, however, when the control I've been keeping over my emotions is ripped from my hands, and my tears rush to break free.

We usually find it comical . . . our intense moments followed by me hiccupping and trying to control the outbursts. This is different, and Jesse holds me tight and rubs my neck as I try to catch my breath.

"I'm fine," I whimper while throwing off the covers and escaping to the bathroom to wash my face.

"You sure?" he asks, and I wave him away. "I'll get you a glass of water."

I splash cold water on my face and hold a wet washcloth to my eyes as I sit down on the toilet in the dark bathroom. I don't need to go, but I can't return to bed yet. I am incapacitated by everything spilling out of me. I'm grateful for the washcloth that soaks up the tears that won't stop streaming. I begin to hold my breath, hoping to calm myself.

"Feeling better?" Jesse asks when he returns with the water. I can't respond and wave him away again. He ignores my gesture, quickly setting the glass on the counter and leaning down to comfort me as best he can in the cramped space. He pushes my hair back, and I simply bury my face further in the washcloth.

"Oh, honey," he whispers and begins to rub my neck again.

I feel like I'm suffocating and struggle to regain control.

Breathe out, sob uncontrollably. "I just . . ."

Breathe out, sob hysterically. ". . . don't know . . ."

Breathe out, sob wildly. ". . . how to live with this."

I doubt Jesse can understand me, but I need to get these thoughts out of my head. I need to free these thoughts and feelings that have been chasing one another inside of me, making me feel frenzied and incapable of handling even the smallest of tasks.

"I know, baby." Jesse wants so desperately to comfort me, to make things right, to bring back all I've lost. Just as my words are drowning in grief, his are cloaked in pain and helplessness. Hearing this breaks my last feeble attempt at self-control.

I moan and howl while he holds me tight.

CHAPTER THIRTY-FOUR

Fall Asleep with Roses in My Hand

Back at the hospital this morning. Breakfast of weak instant oatmeal and a diet Pepsi. Fortifying myself for the day, hoping for a little more change. Seeking answers, but it is evident to me... evident that I don't know what I know, I guess.

I feel myself folding in, creating a cocoon into which I can withdraw in order to sit with my grief. To finally experience the pain and attempt to process it appropriately so I can reach the other side in a better position than I was when we started this journey.

Each day dawns with new hope and possibility. Me determined to do better, be better, and earn the kudos sent my way. Then we become busy with therapies and the routine of hospital life, and by midafternoon I'm flailing about. Unable to capture my anger or reel in my impatience.

I disappoint myself on a daily basis.

My ability to recover is diminishing.

Today, I started having morbid thoughts.

The thoughts crept in while walking Jessica to her room after morning therapy. I let them sit for a minute, trying not to deny them, practicing new theories from sessions with David, hoping they will be easier to process if I'm not in a state of denial. Also, I hoped by going through the motions of getting Jessica to the room and into bed, putting on a movie or some music, having visitors and in-room music, plus Reiki therapy... I thought the activity would take over, and I would be able to brush the thoughts aside.

It hasn't happened yet.

I'm in the process of getting Jessica cleaned up and dressed for her afternoon therapy, and I keep having to stop to take a breath and fight the tears that threaten to fall.

This avalanche of thoughts began with one slippery little thought: *I wonder how things would have been if Jessica hadn't survived her accident.*

One thought. That's all my imagination and raw emotions needed. Before I knew it, details of the memorial service were playing in my mind: dozens of roses and daisies, the music, the slideshow, the people who would attend.

I couldn't stop there, though. I had to wonder what things would be like after.

I imagined lying on the couch, holding Jocelyn tight, zoning out while she watches a movie.

I imagined sitting in the middle of Jessica's bedroom, crying as I packed up all of her possessions, trying to decide what to keep for Jocelyn, what to give to others, and what to keep forever.

The people who might surround us afterward, those whose presence I would be grateful for and those I would resent for their need to make our family's tragedy about themselves. Those who would use the accident as fodder for gossip versus those who actually care.

The tears come when realization sets in.

It is exactly what I am experiencing right now.

My grief is not gentle with me.

When I was sixteen years old, I saw my first psychic at a carnival in Oregon. When I say "saw her," I don't mean that I merely passed by her booth, thinking, *Huh, psychic.* No, I went in, paid my money, and had a reading done. I don't remember too much about that reading except for one thing: She told me that I would have three children.

Over the years, I've been somewhat of a sucker for psychics or whatever it is that they choose to call themselves (intuitive readers, channelers, mediums, clairvoyants, etc.). I definitely believe in other realms and that we all have the ability to see more than meets the eye. So I suppose I would be considered an easy mark.

The three-children thing is a theme that ran consistent in most of the readings I have received throughout my life. It could be very disconcerting, especially during the years when I didn't plan to have any children at all. At one point, one woman (a gypsy, if I recall correctly) got more specific and foretold: "Not three children; three pregnancies." While somewhat troubling, it did make more sense at that point in my life.

Yet here we are, present day, and I have had four pregnancies. I have only given birth to two daughters, and Jesse, to whom I am happily married, has... well, let's just say we won't be able to get pregnant again. Three children. Three pregnancies. I thought they were all wrong.

Until now.

On April 29, 2010, I lost my first-born child. She may not have died, but the child that she was is gone. Even if Jessica achieves what her doctors, therapists, and/or family consider to be a full recovery, it will take several years, and I don't believe she will be exactly as she was.

I realize that none of us is the same person we were when we were ten years old, but the changes that happen are slow, and most parents are given the luxury of gradual changes over several years.

The Jessica we raised for ten years was lost to us suddenly and tragically, and while shades of her former self shine through, the further she progresses in her admittedly miraculous recovery, the more we find she has changed.

In that sense, I will live this life having raised three children. Jessica pre-accident, Jocelyn, and Jessica post-accident.

It is one of the hardest things to convey to people. It is a miracle that Jessica is alive. It is a miracle that she is in the bed beside me, moving, breathing, living, and recovering. But she is not the Jessica I lived with, raised, and grew to love with all of my being.

While there are shades of Jessica's pre-accident personality present, I feel I have lost Pre-Accident Jessica forever, and that fills me with grief and sorrow that feel impossible to navigate.

I don't understand how I am supposed to interact with Post-Accident Jessica. Right now I am angry with her and resent her for taking my baby girl from me.

I have had three children.

Those fucking psychics were right.

I choke back tears, open my computer, and send a message to Jesse.

Maybe I should go on meds. Nothing is working. I prepare myself for being here, prepared to do what needs to be done, be positive about all she's doing, yadda yadda yadda, yet I can't stand this! I cannot stand being here. I cannot stand the never-ending bullshit of this situation. Gah, and I'm doing it again. Complaining to you when you're working your ass off to support us and make things better. I'm sorry. I need to figure this situation out. I need to figure it out, because I can't go on like this.

It's okay, honey. I agree, though. We've got to figure out a way to sort this out for you. When you're away from the hospital, it doesn't really seem to help your mood.

No, because I have to come back. I'm so sick of this. I hate our life.

You have to figure out a way to accept it. You have to figure out how to accept HER. I think it has been easier for me than you, for obvious reasons—you are much more connected to the "old" Jessica than I. The situation, location, daily routine/necessities, all the crap is really second to accepting her as she is. No matter how well we work out the other parts of our life, nothing will truly help you get through this until you accept Jessica as she is. You have to figure that part out. She's not her old self and may never be. She is, however, still our daughter. Despite all the negative aspects of her injury and its impact, she is full of light and joy. It's not the same as old Jessica, but it is similar in many ways. I think you will have to choose to accept that and live with it, or you will end up abandoning her.

Yeah, that is the major problem. I just can't. I haven't even had the chance to grieve for the old Jessica. I can't accept this new Jessica yet. This grief is so fresh and new. How am I supposed to handle it?

I understand, honey. It is hard to let go of the past, especially when you were so, SO connected to the old Jessica. If and when you find a way to do it, I think you will find the new Jessica is quite lovely. She's constantly regaining the ability to be the old Jessica. Only time will tell how much of that she can regain, but part of the recovery has to come from us. If we can't be committed to helping the new Jessica, we risk stalling the transition to her old self. Or whatever the transition could be. Anyway, that's how I see it. I'm sorry it's so hard, baby. I'm here for you, if there is anything I can do that you think would help. I love you.

I don't see her as lovely, though. That's the problem. She is all parts of a child, any child, I resent. She doesn't listen to us or the therapists; she is mean; she does rude things intentionally. I had no patience for that type of behavior before the accident, let alone now. What you're saying is 100 percent correct. I don't have it in me. Like I said, I keep trying to build myself up. I keep trying to get there... and when I return, it's worse. I keep thinking it will be better, but it's not. It's just not, and I can't act like I don't understand why. Because my Jessica is gone. I'm sorry, honey. This isn't the sort of thing you want to hear from the mother of your children. I'm sorry.

Don't apologize. I understand what you're saying. Part of what she needs right now is compassion. I can imagine it's hard for you to give, but when it is given, she responds. I was able to get her to respond and stop pinching over the weekend by talking her through it. It took a lot of work, though, and I get that it's hard for you right now. I guess that's what I meant by the whole acceptance part. I was only able to find the patience with her because I'm beginning to accept her. Until you can do that, it will be very difficult to do anything with her. I'm sorry it's so hard, though. I don't think I can really imagine the pain it causes you.

And that's the problem. If my husband, Jessica's father, who is closest to us and so wise, if he can't understand the level of pain I'm in, who can?

CODA

An invisible thread connects those who are destined to meet, regardless of time, place, and circumstance. The thread may stretch and tangle, but it will never break.

Ancient Chinese Proverb

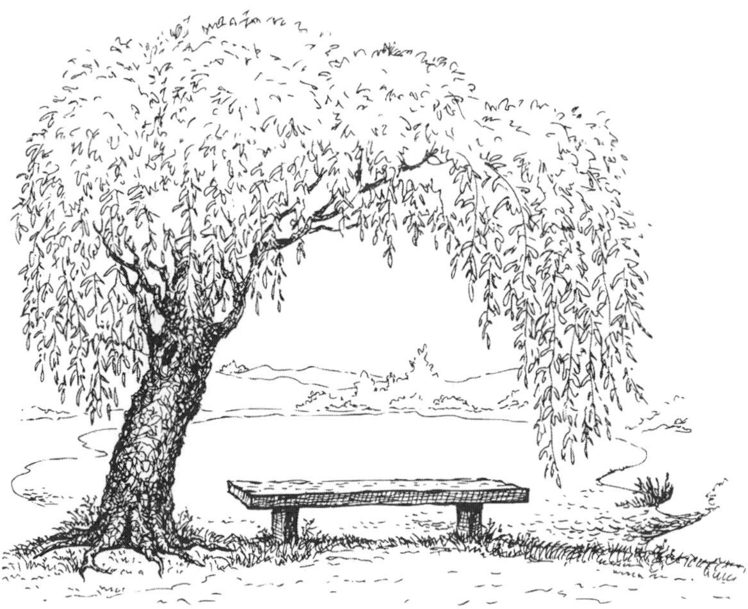

CHAPTER THIRTY-FIVE

Make Our Dreams Come True

"Good morning, Jessica. Jolene." Faye greets us in the hall outside the pediatric therapy gym for our final occupational therapy session for this inpatient rehab stay. After seven weeks, we're getting ready to be discharged. "Are you ready to go home?"

Jessica nods and laughs, and I smile at Faye. "Yes. It's been great, and she's made some good progress, but it will definitely be nice to have our family all under one roof again."

"Sure thing."

"Okay, girl, what'll it be today?" Faye wheels Jessica over to the game cabinet and opens the doors. I'm still amazed at Jessica's newfound ability to lean forward and point to a box.

"Buckaroo Bonzai it is." Faye grabs the box and wheels Jessica to the mat with the table in front of it. I sit in the chair across the room to disturb their session as little as possible.

I only sit in on about half of the therapy sessions these days. Jessica seems to "perform" better for the therapists when I'm not there, but I still like to see what she's doing. It also allows me to talk to the therapists about her progress and exercises, get advice, and basically indulge in adult interaction while stuck in the hospital.

When I sit in, however, I make it a point to have a book, paperwork, or my phone with me so I can feign interest in something else instead of making Jessica feel like I am watching her the entire time. Today is no different.

I try to check email and Facebook on my phone but keep being distracted by the squeals of Jessica's laughter and the noise from their activity. I put my phone in my pocket and watch Faye and Jessica interact.

Buckaroo Bonzai involves a horse on a stand and a bunch of plastic pieces to hang on him. Things like a rope, a saddle, and a horseshoe. I'm not surprised Jessica chose this game, because it's *Toy Story* themed and the horse is Woody's pal Bullseye. Both Pre-Accident and Post-Accident Jessica can watch the *Toy Story* movies over and over again.

I am, however, a bit horrified by the game itself. You have to be careful when hanging the plastic pieces on the horse, because if you bump him too much, he will start bucking, and all of the pieces will go flying. This is the part that cracks Jessica up the most, as it means Faye has to try to stop the pieces from landing on the floor.

Faye sets up the horse, and they carefully place all the pieces. Then Jessica purposely bumps Bullseye, and Faye scrambles for flying cowboy parts while Jessica turns red with laughter.

It's a little funny ha-ha and a little funny uh-oh, but it turns into a little funny stop-my-heart-and-help-me-not-break-down on their final turn. Jessica sends the pieces flying and looks up at me, points to the back foot of the horse, and then points to her head. All the while cracking up.

Faye and I look at each other, eyes wide.

"At least she's got a good attitude about it," Faye says softly.

"Yeah," I whisper as they start to clean up.

"Hi, Jessica!" Trish comes through the door.

Before Faye leaves, she leans down to give me a quick hug and an apologetic look. "So sorry about that," she whispers in my ear.

I shake my head and reply, "Not your fault."

I pull my phone out to text Jesse and share this story with him immediately.

Trish leaves Jessica on the mat to continue working on her sitting balance. I occupy myself throughout their session until, again, I hear Jessica giggling.

"Hey, Mom, I thinks she's trying to get your attention," Trish says.

I look up to see Jessica giggling through her look-what-I-can-do smile. "What is it, honey?"

She and Trish both look down at Jessica's feet. I follow their gaze, gasp, and call in a broken voice, "First position!"

"She did that on her own," Trish says, and Jessica giggles some more and tries to raise her hands above her head.

"Sunshine arms?" I ask her. More giggles. Her body is bent over, and her arms only make it to forehead level due to her restricted range of motion, but I am still overwhelmed by the effect dance has had on her recovery. It is a magical sight to see.

Ann enters the gym, and Trish transfers Jessica into her wheelchair. "Are you guys staying in here?"

"No, we'll go over to the speech room." Ann grabs Jessica's chair and pushes her down the short hallway and into a small room across from the peds gym.

The speech room is better suited than the gym for the work the speech therapists do with Jessica. We settle into our chairs and are joined by two interns who shadow the speech therapists a couple of days a week.

"Are you all ready to head home?" Ann repeats the familiar question, and Jessica smiles at her. "We'll have an easy day, Jessica. We've pushed you hard enough in the past few weeks."

She sits across the desk from Jessica and fires up the computer. "Let's see what we've got."

Upon discovering Jessica's love of music, the speech therapists began incorporating YouTube videos into Jessica's sessions. They made a deal with her that if she works on an assignment for an allotted period of time, she can pick a music video to watch for thirty seconds to a minute as a reward.

As a treat today, Ann begins the session this way. "What would you like to listen to, Jessica?"

Jessica turns on her iPad, opens the ProLoQ app, pushes the music category, and selects her choice.

Sara Bareilles, her robotic voice commands.

"Good choice," I whisper.

Ann types Jessica's selection into the search bar on YouTube and then moves the monitor closer to Jessica so she can select the video she wants to watch.

"Good choice," I repeat as Jessica points to the screen. Ann clicks the mouse, and the familiar piano notes fill the air.

Something always brings me back to you… I lean into Jessica, and she pushes her head towards me. I melt into her beautiful eyes and continue to sing. *It never takes too long; no matter what I say or do, I'll still feel you here 'til the moment I'm gone…*

It's difficult to sing my favorite lines in such a small office, especially since Jessica and I now have our foreheads pressed together. It's just another thirty seconds or so, though, so I press on.

Set me free, leave me be. I don't wanna fall another moment into your gravity…

As the music plays on and Jessica reaches out to squeeze my hand, it becomes increasingly difficult to contain the emotion I'm usually free to release when belting out this song. Why isn't Ann turning it off?

You loved me 'cause I'm fragile, but I thought that I was strong. You touch me for a little while, and all my fragile strength is gone…

I close my eyes and try to regulate my breathing through the remainder of the song, singing lower than is intended for this powerful ballad.

I live here on my knees, as I try to make you see that you're everything I think I need here on the ground…

A deep breath through the glory note, and I reopen my eyes to sing directly to Jess.

Something always brings me back to you; it never takes too long. I finish singing and kiss her on the forehead. We turn to face Ann and the interns to find them all wiping their eyes and laughing softly.

One starts. "That was..."

The other finishes. "Amazing?"

"Did you pick that for me?" I ask Jess, and she nods.

"I love you, Peanut Butter."

She squeezes my hand again.

CHAPTER THIRTY-SIX

Live as One

December 15, 2010

"Hey, guys." Holly enters the room with her ever-present stack of paperwork. "Are you ready to go?"

Grateful for the break in packing up the hospital room, I sit down to chat with her. "I hope so. You're probably the fifteenth person to ask us that today."

"Well, I know everyone will miss you, but we're very excited for Jessica to get home and continue working hard in outpatient therapy."

"Oh, yeah, is that set up yet?"

"Yes, that's part of the discharge paperwork the nurses will have for you. I believe the inpatient therapists actually called last week in order to get Jessica on the schedule without too much of a wait."

"Oh, great. I was worried about her having a break in therapy."

"It shouldn't be too bad. So what about you and Jesse? Are you glad to be home for the holidays? Do you have any big plans once you get home?"

I look at Jessica in the bed and shake my head. Pretty much every holiday or birthday that has occurred since her accident has been spent in the hospital, so many of the events we attended or traditions we had were lost. Hospital life lends itself to a great time distortion, making it difficult to grasp that the holiday season is already upon us.

"I don't know. We'll see how we feel when we get home and settle into a routine. I know it's not possible for life to get back to normal, but finding a new state of normal would be nice."

"It seems to me that you and Jesse have done a great job of adapting to the changes in your life."

"That's because you're not privy to our bluntly honest and heartbreaking discussions."

"Of course."

"I've been pretty whiny lately. I think the shock of the accident is finally starting to wear off. My depression and grief have been overwhelming."

"Are you getting help?" Holly leans forward, a look of concern on her face.

"Yes. I started seeing a therapist."

"How's that going?"

"Oh, it's going. He's helping me honestly address the things I'm feeling."

"That's good, because you're dealing with a lot."

I sigh and roll my eyes. "I know, but how long can 'dealing with a lot' be an excuse?" I look out the window, gathering my thoughts. "It's funny. One of my core beliefs is in the power of the written and spoken word, specifically that thoughts become our reality."

"Okay," Holly says to indicate she's following along.

"Well, a few weeks ago, Jesse and I had a pretty depressing conversation in which I told him that I hate our life. If I believe our words matter, I need to be consistent, both intellectually and spiritually, and try to live that belief in every situation."

"How do you mean?"

"If I judge myself and think I'm handling our situation wrong, then I shouldn't be hurt and surprised when others judge me, as well. I don't get to moan and groan about how hard my life is and how much I hate it and then wonder when it's going to change and why The Universe keeps piling crap on."

"Right, but... it's a difficult situation."

"Oh, I agree with that. I will proudly wear my Captain Obvious hat and honestly and vehemently say with 100 percent authority that this situation sucks. I've described it best as mind-numbing, heartbreaking, and soul-crushing. I am dependent on things I can't change and powerless in such a way that I generally feel useless, but there's one person who has it worse than me."

She glances at my daughter, who is lying in the bed, playing on her iPad, and I nod.

"Talk about being at the mercy of things you can't control. And what does she do for most of her days? She laughs. She smiles at us and laughs at our lame jokes and works on moving her body as much as she can. She is fighting every minute of every day to get back to us. Seven weeks of inpatient rehab later, it hasn't been completely easy—"

Holly interrupts. "Would that be an understatement?"

"Of the century," I say, confirming her assumption. "For sure. But I'm proud of Jessica and the progress she's made. For a kid who could have had seizures, never moved the left side of her body, and possibly been blind, all as a result of the accident? I'd say she's doing pretty well."

Holly looks at Jessica again. "Many of the things we take for granted, she has spent almost two months relearning."

"I won't claim it's easy. Our journey continues, and she still has a long way to go, but I could take a lesson from her in maintaining a good attitude through a challenging situation."

"We all could." Holly calls over to Jessica, "You're pretty amazing, kid."

Jessica moves her eyes between the two of us, grins, and says, "Uh-huh."

As I continue to pack up the room, I think about Holly's original question: "What are your plans for the holidays?"

When I was a kid, Christmas Day was a huge production. Even in the years when we were warned that "Christmas is going to be tight," we'd wake up on Christmas morning to piles of presents under the tree.

The traditions of stockings hung with care, chocolate for breakfast, finding the perfect place to sit, and matching Santa gifts to the recipients followed me while growing up.

However, for all the energy we put into Christmas, I don't remember going to church very often. We were too busy with gifts, meeting up with extended family, and meal preparation. As a result, when I grew older and started examining my own beliefs, I realized the "Reason for the Season" wasn't even something we celebrated, and I began feeling uneasy about the excessive celebrations. I worked hard to put my own traditions in place and create new traditions for my children.

We exchange our family gifts on Winter Solstice, the longest night of the year. We honor the change of the season and the returning of the light. We developed our own tradition of cinnamon rolls for breakfast, a fire in the fireplace, and the exchanging of a few special gifts. We top off the day with a nice dinner.

We refer to Christmas as Santa Day, when the girls receive one or two bigger gifts from the jolly old soul. It's been perfect. Before tragedy struck, I'd planned to add more experiences to our box of traditions.

No matter what the celebration entails, it's hard to plan if the Spirit is elusive.

Solstice falls on a Tuesday this year, and being in the hospital means Jesse and I haven't had a chance to plan meals and gifts or do any shopping. Jesse also has to work that day, so our evening will likely be rushed.

It's hard not to lament the loss of new traditions, such as heading to Tahoe for a few days so Jesse could share his love of skiing with

Jessica while Jocelyn and I built snowmen and had snowball fights. Or taking the entire family to see *The Nutcracker* performed by the Sacramento Ballet.

Instead of giving Jessica her usual Big Box O'Books, I will concentrate on board games and craft activities that will double as therapy. Thankfully, Jocelyn is young enough to be enchanted by "Lights! Snowman!," so I'm sure she will enjoy whatever we do.

Perhaps I should simply look forward to our much-needed time together as a family. Jessica and I have been in the hospital for seven weeks. Jesse has come to stay occasionally, but 98 percent of the therapy, movies, AFO management, doctors' rounds, conversations with nurses, meltdowns, cafeteria food, meditation, lost holidays, and hoped-for progress have been me and Jessica. I don't know how we kept from going crazy.

This hospital stay has been more hopeful and optimistic than our first stay directly after the accident, when we focused on bringing Jessica back from death's door. Still, these special living arrangements have taken their toll on our family.

All of our relationships are so strained that I will be grateful to be home and have our baking day with Kari and Hannah and sit in front of the fire drinking hot chocolate and watching cheesy holiday movies, all while we continue to do what we do.

We can do away with the gifts and fanfare, because, more than anything, I'd like to receive Peace. I want to be able to calm my mind and my heart. I want my anger and grief to dissipate and the love and joy to overwhelm me again.

Letting go of the resentment I have toward those who have hurt our family since Jessica's accident and, instead, concentrating on the love that surrounds us would be the greatest gift. I want to once again accept Jessica's survival for the miracle it is, regardless of where she is in her recovery.

I want to remember how to simply be.

CHAPTER THIRTY-SEVEN

Can't Keep Waiting to Live

January

"Happy New Year, honey!" Jesse makes a point of kissing me deeply at midnight. The girls are in bed, and our New Year's Eve celebration has involved sharing a bottle of wine on the couch while we watch some of the shows that have built up on our DVR over the past seven weeks.

"Mmm, happy New Year." I snuggle closer to him and unpause the show.

"This will be a better year. Jessica's doing well. I feel like we can finally get to work on getting back to normal."

I pause the show again and lean forward to put my wine glass on the table. "Do you really think so?" I ask. The words are barely able to leave my mouth under the weight of doubt that hangs from each of them.

"I do. Yeah. You said her outpatient therapy is progressing well, didn't you? She's working hard to increase the strength in the rest of her body. They're helping her with all of the skills she needs to live independently again."

"Yeah, but…" We're several months into therapy now and two weeks out from Jessica's inpatient rehab stay, and I'm still fighting to walk the line between grieving and recovery. I try to choose my words carefully, not wanting to start an argument or burst Jesse's optimistic bubble.

"I'm not sure that's realistic," I state simply.

"What isn't? Her living independently?"

"Yes." The cloud of doom rushes into the room, and I take a deep breath and exhale, trying to blow it away. "No. I don't know. I think..." I grab my wine and drain the glass.

Jesse reasons with me. "Well, it won't happen tomorrow; I know that."

"I know, but okay. Here's what I mean. This week at the outpatient clinic, they had scheduled her sessions so we had a big break between occupational and speech therapy."

"Okay." Jesse studies the floor as he listens.

"She had PT first, physically tiring. OT next, both physically and mentally tiring. Then we went to the cafeteria to have lunch before her ST appointment."

As I outline the day for him more clearly, understanding creeps onto Jesse's face. "Which means by the time speech rolls around, she's pretty tired from all the other therapies and being in the wheelchair for so long."

"Exactly. The outpatient speech therapist, Michelle, ran some language tests to get a baseline of Jess's cognition, and even though it wasn't the full test and we don't have the results yet, I was sitting in on the appointment and following along with the test. Jessica wasn't doing well. I actually asked Michelle to cut the test short and try again next week, when the schedule is reversed and speech is first rather than last. Thankfully, she agreed."

"Well, that's good."

"You're right. Unless she wasn't just tired."

"What do you mean?"

"What if we go to the appointment next week, and she tests the same as she did this week? What if she has the processing and expressive deficits these tests check for? Even if she doesn't, the fact that she can't go past noon in her wheelchair, undergoing different therapies and activities, without it affecting her ability to take a test like this could affect other things. Like when she gets to go back to school and what school looks like when she goes back."

I stand up to take my wine glass to the kitchen. I'm not sure if I'm going to refill it or put it in the sink. I'll decide when I get there.

Jesse follows me. "So, you believe she's done recovering, then?"

I pause, hang my head, and then refill the glass. I take a drink before responding. "No, I don't. I still believe in her ability to recover, but there is a long way to go. And 'a long way to go' doesn't refer only to how much potential she has to recover and all of the ways she still can and will recover but also to the time frame we are in now."

Jesse leans against the counter, crosses his arms, and nods along with what I'm saying. "So..."

I close my eyes and try to remember why we got into this conversation in the first place. It's certainly not the way I'd have picked to start our new year.

"I think," I say slowly, "we need to stop. I can't talk anymore. About any of it. It hasn't even been a year since her accident. Can we let go of the idea of independence and normal and dreams of being able to go to Monterey or Disneyland or ever being able to do anything like that again? For now, anyway. I can't talk about any of it anymore. Let's focus on being a family. Let's go back to doing family stuff. Let's have regular days with a kid who has special needs. With a disabled child. I can't talk anymore about treatments and insurance and trying to fix the things that might not ever be able to be fixed. Let's just be a family."

"Of course we can." Jesse steps closer to my side of the kitchen to take me in his arms. "Of course we are."

"Recovery is too much," I mumble against his chest. "We're trying to have a normal life, but recovery interferes with normal." I push away from him. "And who said we were guaranteed normal anyway? Everyone has tragedy. Everyone has their own battles. We had ours before; we'll have more in the future. It's just life, and trying to fix it away, trying to talk it away, trying to make it all go back to the way it was can't be the right way to handle things. Let's spend this year trying to move forward."

He takes our wine glasses and puts them in the sink and then starts turning out the lights in the house. "That sounds like a good plan to me."

"Okay, I know we've only been at this for a few months now, but I'm pretty sure I had a breakthrough the other night."

"Oh?" Each visit with David leaves me feeling more comfortable in sharing the ups and downs of my days with him.

"Yeah. On New Year's Eve, Jesse and I had a big discussion about…" I try to distill my conversation with Jesse into one word. "A normal life."

"Oh? That sounds interesting."

"If you want to call it that." I briefly recap our family's holiday message for him.

"So what was the breakthrough then?"

"I don't know how to explain it. It's kind of exhausting." I go over the conversation with Jesse in my mind and what I feel has changed since then.

"Is it…" David tries to ask a question that will help me clarify my thoughts. "Is it being able to have a conversation about moving forward?"

I consider this for a minute. "I suppose that's part of it. And not. It's all of it." I throw my hands up. "Every day is like a tightrope. Half the time I'm excited about the progress Jessica is making, and half the time the grief is still coming in waves."

"How do you keep from going under?" he asks.

"I don't know that I do," I admit. "Every day, whether I mean to or not, the memory of her lying in the dirt with her head split open appears in my head. The last time I saw her whole and the first time I saw her so broken. Each day further from the accident is both harder and easier in her recovery."

He studies me for a minute, and I concentrate on clarifying myself again.

"I know. Imagine living it. It's impossible. She almost died..." My voice catches, and I grab the box of tissues off the bookshelf before he has the chance to push them toward me. "She almost died. Had the impact been half an inch in any other direction, she would not have lived. Had the ambulance taken a split second longer to respond, she would not have lived. Had the trauma doctors hesitated any longer, she would not have lived. If the neuro team at UCD hadn't put the drain into her head the following day, she wouldn't have lived.

"It is a miracle that she survived this horrible accident, and I am in awe and humbled by that."

"But?"

"But we can't go back to how things were. Even if she has a full recovery, she will be different. Changed. And waiting for that to happen? Waiting for recovery and being in denial of the fact that she is not recovered now? Waiting for her to recover before we move forward with life won't work. Denying the fact that she is disabled, handicapped, special needs is a way of denying who she is now. It denies her services and keeps me in a place where I am not moving forward but am being stagnant, wallowing in my own misery. That doesn't do me any good."

We sit in silence for a moment. I can almost see my words dancing on the air, spinning around the sacred space of his office, enjoying their freedom from the cage I've kept them in for so long.

He speaks first. "I think you're right."

"What? I am? About what?"

"I'd definitely call that a breakthrough."

February

"Hey, honey, are you planning to change?" I'm sitting at the table, playing UNO with Jessica, when Jesse comes into the room.

"Are you talking to me?" I look at him, confused, as I lay down a green seven.

"Yes, I'm talking to you."

Two months out of inpatient rehab and our family is starting to settle into a routine. Jesse and I are both relieved that we are able to do more things for ourselves instead of relying on the kindness of our friends, our family, and strangers. Today, on a not-so-rare warm February day, we spent some time cleaning up our backyard while Jocelyn ran around with Sugar and Jessica watched it all from the patio.

When we came in, we showered off the dirt and grime, but unlike me, Jesse is dressed in slacks and a button-down shirt. I'm wearing comfy clothes for a Saturday evening at home. I look at him dumbly before asking, "What are you talking about?"

"Jessica, I want to take your mom out for Valentine's Day tonight. Will you be okay to watch your sister on your own?"

Jessica looks at Jocelyn, who is coloring at her art table, glances back at her dad, and then pulls the iPad closer and starts typing. Jesse mouths at me to "go get dressed," but I'm eager to see what Jessica is spending so much time typing. I hand him my UNO cards so he can take over for me and then lean over to watch the words form on Jessica's screen. She completes her sentence and hits Speak with a grin.

I was going to say everything but the diapers, but she's not wearing diapers anymore, so okay, that's fine.

Jesse and I burst out laughing, and he motions again for me to get dressed.

"Do we need to get the girls ready, too? Are they coming with us?"

"Gah, if you must know, Kari and Hannah are coming over. Now, please. Go get dressed. They'll be here soon."

Hearing this news, Jessica starts laughing and dancing in her wheelchair. I guess Jesse doesn't need to bother to clear the rest of the plan with her. She approves.

As I hurry to the bedroom to change my clothes and put on some makeup, I consider what Jessica said about babysitting Jocelyn. The fact that she can't walk or talk didn't enter her mind. What she thought would keep her from babysitting her sister is the fact that she doesn't want to change a poopy diaper. Anything else she can handle, regardless of circumstance.

Her determination and spirit are qualities I need to remember when I'm whining about the pile of paperwork I have to shuffle through for taxes or arguing with the insurance company about her services.

March

I creep into Jessica's bedroom on the morning of her birthday and crawl into bed beside her. She's already awake and turns to smile at me.

"Good morning, good morning; it's a great day to be alive. Good morning, good morning to you, you, a boo ba di do. Good morning, good morning; it's a great day to be alive. Good morning, good morning to you.

"I love you, Jessica. Happy birthday, my Sweetest Pete."

She laughs at my song, and my eyes are wet with tears as I remember the last time I sang this song to her, almost a year ago.

Jessica smiles at me and holds up her left hand, twisting it back and forth. She looks at it in amazement and then back at me.

"Oh, did it suddenly start working again?"

She nods, with a big grin, showing me how she can splay out her fingers flatter than she has been able to do until now.

"Great job, honey! What a great birthday present."

We snuggle up for a bit as I stall the process of getting us both up and ready for our day.

CHAPTER THIRTY-EIGHT

Of Melodies Pure and True

April 29, 2011 – One Year Later

"Hey, Jessica." Dr. Manhart enters the exam room and shakes Jessica's shoulder a bit before sitting down at the computer and signing on.

Jessica laughs and types on her iPad, and the robotic voice issues forth: *Hi, Larry.*

"Jessica! Sorry, Dr. Manhart." I apologize through my laughter, but "Larry" is unfazed.

"Hey, that's pretty cool." He rolls over to look at Jessica's iPad, and she shows off the icons for him.

My name is Jessica. I am eleven years old. My favorite color is orange. Do you want to play UNO?

"Well, all right!" Manhart rolls back over to the computer and types in some notes. "When did she get this fancy contraption?"

"While we were in inpatient rehab in December. She's doing really well on it."

"Do you want to play UNO?" Jessica repeats.

"Ha ha. No thank you, girlfriend. We'll play when we get home."

"And how is outpatient therapy progressing? How is she doing?"

The appointment is similar in flow to the first appointment we had with Dr. Manhart after we changed insurance months ago, except in the progress Jessica has made and the abilities she is able to display.

The team of outpatient therapists is building her strength on the parallel bars and with a walker. She is practicing her ADLs, which are activities for daily living, and is increasing her range of motion and getting faster at dressing herself and brushing her own teeth and hair.

She is still not speaking and has issues with her secretion management, which may take the longest to correct.

Life is simultaneously easier and harder now. We are able to do more "normal" things as a family, like shopping or attending birthday parties, but the level of care she needs is more involved than ever before. We are on the move from the moment we wake up in the morning until we fall into bed at night.

Jessica is exerting her independence and wants to do more physically, eat more foods, visit more places, and continue to move down the path of recovery. She is determined.

I relay everything to Dr. Manhart as he does his physical exam of Jessica. He tests her reflexes and takes off the AFOs to check her spasticity. He even brings in a walker and asks her to show how far she is able to ambulate with it.

"This is all great news. She's continuing to do very well," he comments as he continues to type the results of his exam into the computer. "Questions?"

"Um, yes. Today's the day, isn't it?" I look at him expectantly.

He checks the computer and looks at me again, a little confused. "What day?"

"One year later. We were told way back when that today is the magic day. Today you would be able to tell us how much she will be able to recover or where she will be in the future."

"I can't tell you that."

My shoulders slump, and I cock my head like a dog that wants something it can't have. "But—"

"I'm sorry, but there is no magic day. Especially not when Jessica continues to make progress every time I see her. As long as she's progressing, anything is possible. Let's set her up to come back in three months, and we'll talk again then." He stands and grabs the discharge paperwork off the printer and hands the forms to me. "Anything else?"

I start to look through the papers, hoping to find the answers I've been seeking for 365 days. They're not in there.

"No. Thank you, Dr. Manhart. We'll see you in three months."

"Well, that's a good thing," Jesse says to reassure me after I tell him about the specifics of the appointment when the four of us are home that evening.

"How so? I've been looking forward to this day for a year, hoping to get answers. Hoping to know more."

"Honey..." He takes my hand gently. "Do you really want him to tell you now, when Jessica is eleven years old, what she will be capable of when she's twenty? Or thirty? Or sixty? Or would you rather have a future full of possibilities?"

CHAPTER THIRTY-NINE

Whisper Words of Wisdom

"Where does your serenity come from?"

I'm sitting on the leather couch in David's office. When he asks this question, I slowly close my eyes and take a deep breath.

"I don't know if I'd call what I'm feeling *serenity*. It feels more like defeat. I feel defeated."

David's eyebrows shoot up. Apparently this isn't the answer he was expecting. "Defeated by what? What have you lost?"

"Everything." I sigh and stare at the *Serenity Road*, one of the pieces of art that hangs on the wall behind him, while trying to dissect my feelings further in order to express them accurately. I realized long ago that if I am paying for my therapy out of pocket, no good can come from lying about what I'm feeling or how I'm coping or from claiming how perfect and rosy my life is. If I'm shelling out $110.00 a session, I'm going to get my money's worth. I'm determined to be fixed, dammit.

"I guess I never really thought about the use of the word *defeat* before." I begin to make circular motions in front of my chest, fingers pointed in, as if I am trying to clear away the thick layers of skin and muscle to expose the core of my being to this man, only the second one with whom I have shared the ugliest parts of myself. "I just feel empty. Or maybe what you said last week is true. I'm getting better at coping. Oh, also, my period is gone. I don't have to deal with the overwhelming aspects of my days with a surge of hormones rushing through me. But this . . . ," I say, motioning to my chest again, "is the same.

"The heartbreak of Jessica's accident, the hole it caused, and the grief are still there. The vast emptiness of…" I swallow hard and struggle to continue as the tears rise up like a tide greets the shore. "See? If I talk about the specifics long enough and try to articulate them, it all comes out. If I didn't care about being presentable in public, if I didn't care about what people would think, this is how I would walk around all day, every day. Life would be easy. But I can't do that."

"So, that hole, that grief…" He takes a moment to adjust himself in his chair, and I clasp my hands together and bite my lip. If this were a poker game, seat adjustment would be David's "tell." A sign that things are about to get more serious.

He starts gently. "I guess I'm confused. You feel defeated because the grief and emptiness are still there?"

"Yes," I answer quickly before catching myself. "I know that's not fair. I'm aware that Jessica's accident is a huge thing, and the aftermath isn't simply going to go away. I don't feel defeated because the grief is still there; it's more like…" I take a minute of my own to shift my position on the couch. I end up leaning forward, elbows on my knees.

"You said I'm coping better these days, but I'm not sure I am. Part of me agrees with you. I'll be living day to day just fine. So fine, in fact, that you used the word *serenity* to describe it; but then my period hits, and, well, I've been here, so you've seen what happens. I go from *fine* and *serene* to a point where I can't talk without crying.

"I'm frustrated that I'm not better. But even more than that, I'm frustrated by the days when it *seems* like I'm better, it *seems* like I'm coping, when in reality, I'm still in a place of doing what needs to be done, and any minute the smallest and most innocent thing will unseat me, and I'll be drowning again."

I take a breath and look David in the eye. He opens his mouth but closes it without speaking. I lean back on the couch again and wipe my eyes with the edge of my shirt sleeve.

"So, the defeat?"

"The defeat is in the upending, I guess. Feeling like I'm finally handling everything again, and then, oh, look! I'm not. It makes me feel like my only options are to sit and wallow in my grief and depression or robotically go through each day doing what needs to be done. I'm frustrated by those choices. I'd like to move on."

"What would it look like to do more than what needs to be done? What would moving on look like to you?"

I open my mouth to answer and then snap it shut as he did seconds earlier. I rest my head on the back of the couch and study the ceiling. My eyes move from ceiling tile to ceiling tile, air vent to air vent, and light to light. I note the rivets at the intersections and shift my position on the couch again.

"I don't know," I answer honestly. I gesture toward the figurative hole in my chest again. "This feeling hasn't changed since the accident. The pain, the hole, the *loss*. None of it has changed. I think I agree with you. I'm coping better. But these feelings haven't decreased, and I have no idea how to imagine an existence where the hole is not there.

"Moving on would mean... I don't know. Honestly? At this point, I'd simply like to have an easy day."

"And what would *that* look like?"

"An easy day right now would be doing nothing. I could stay in my pajamas, sleep all day, and be red-faced with swollen eyes, letting all of the heartache and depression hang out there in the open without worrying about what anyone thinks."

I meet David's gaze but am overwhelmed by the softness and compassion in his eyes. I study my hands for a minute and then look up. "That's not ideal, and it's certainly not moving on. Moving on, for me, would be actually achieving serenity. An ideal day would be waking up at 5:00 a.m., meditating for an hour, working out, showering, doing my hair and makeup, and helping with the girls. Making them breakfast, doing their hair, and making their lunches for school. Dropping them off, going home, writing, shopping for groceries, preparing dinner, making sure the dishes and laundry are done and the house is picked up..."

The compassion is slowly leaving David's face, and I see a smile forming at the corners of his mouth as I continue with the description of my fantasy world.

"...volunteer...cure cancer...achieve world peace...and have dinner on the table by 5:00."

He chuckles. "So, 1950's Cleaver household or *Father Knows Best*?"

"*Brady Bunch*. Something like that, yeah."

We barely laugh at the absurdity of it. Is he aware that part of me wishes for this fantasy to be real?

"Right. That's ridiculous, but the general idea is there. I'd like to have time to take care of myself and my family in a healthy way. I'd like to contribute, to make things easier on Jesse and be there for my girls."

"That doesn't happen now?"

"Not nearly enough or as easily as I'd like it to. It's a struggle. A *big* struggle. I do what needs to be done, because I can't just sit and wallow. That'd be easy but less than ideal. I want to move on. I want to accept this life that we are living now. I want to let go of the life I thought we would live so I can step into the one we are meant to live."

Meant to live.

I close my eyes.

With those three words, I am back in the Great Unknown with Jessica, planning this incarnation. I take another deep breath. Finally, serenity descends upon me.

I reluctantly leave the safety of David's office and slowly make my way home. I try to concentrate on the road ahead, but my thoughts are pulled, over and over, back to the Great Unknown.

From the moment Jessica's accident happened, I have been

picking points of light out from the darkness. I feel grateful I was the one who took her to her lesson (I wasn't always). I feel grateful Jocelyn fell asleep on the way to the barn (she didn't always), because if she hadn't, we wouldn't have stayed. I feel grateful that the fire department was literally thirty seconds away and responded in just about that long. And, obviously, I have been offering up my appreciation to The Universe for the skilled hands and heads of the doctors, surgeons, and nurses at Sutter Roseville and UC Davis Medical Center.

From the second I came through the gate at the barn and saw Jessica lying on the ground, from the second I slid onto the ground next to her, from the second I could see exactly how bad it was, the only thing I could hear were the Angels I have believed in for so long. All I could hear were their voices in my head, saying, "She will be fine, she will be fine, she will be fine."

It was overwhelming to see exactly how far the Love traveled to help lift up her name and body for healing. Entire schools and churches praying for her; bells being rung in Thailand; candles being lit in Australia, Canada, and England. Her name being spoken in Japan, Sweden, Germany, and Spain. Every state in the U.S. being on board to help her heal.

People dreaming about her whole, recovered, dancing in pink tutus, and running with flowers in her "Sonya hair."

I have never stopped believing she will be fine, but it took a long time before I allowed myself to consider exactly how long the journey would be. I was ignorant about the whole process and didn't think beyond the four-to-six-week time frame they said we would be in the hospital.

I foolishly sent out emails saying, "See you next month."

I believed she would be able to appear on stage and take her own curtsy for her award at her last recital.

I told the cheerleading camp, "We'll have to wait and see if she'll be there at the end of July."

As my eyes were opened by research, doctors, and anecdotal stories, I began to get angry. Angry at the fact that I couldn't do much more than sit there and be angry. The philosophies and beliefs I held that got me through the initial crisis were stretched thin and started to snap.

Through those beliefs, my positive attitude, the magic we created in a worldwide upsurge of love for Jessica, and the sheer force of my (and everyone else's) belief in the thought *she is going to be fine*, I thought we would create miracles, and I'd have my Hollywood moment.

I curse my Great Unknown self for laughing so arrogantly at the lack of real challenges I'd encountered in my past lives. This challenge and these lessons are no joke.

There are definitely lessons I am here to learn this time around; sometimes I feel like I am failing the class. I also feel that Jessica's recovery is dependent upon how well I accept this situation and begin to learn the lessons I outlined for myself.

I'm aware that's a ridiculous notion.

Even though our paths are intertwined, given that we chose one another as mother and daughter, Jessica's recovery is her own doing. Our paths may intersect, run parallel, and be on the same course many times throughout our lives, but they are our individual paths. I need to be wary of falling into the trap of believing the speed at which I master my lessons will directly affect her recovery. She has her own challenges to overcome and lessons to learn.

Mastering my lessons will likely make it *easier* for her to move along her path, as we will both meet with less resistance, anger, resentment, and sadness. Even though our lessons are our own, the despair I feel is so far-reaching. I would be naïve to believe it doesn't affect her on some level.

Getting control of myself and truly concentrating on and mastering things like Patience, Acceptance, Faith, and Trust helps move both of us along our paths. If nothing else, it will help us regain and maintain the Grace with which we were handling this situation in the initial days of crisis.

Given that, I have come to terms with how this happened. This journey has helped me solidify my beliefs. I haven't had a change of heart; I haven't come to Jesus; I haven't apologized to God for not believing. I still believe, as I did before the accident, that we pick our paths before we are born. Jessica and I chose this. If it is not exactly what happened, it's pretty damn close.

If her Traumatic Brain Injury hadn't come from a horse kicking her, it would've been a car accident, a fall from climbing a tree, or some other hurricane sweeping through our lives.

I find the greatest peace when I think about that party in the Great Unknown. I do believe it had to have been a party. Jessica and I couldn't have been the only souls discussing this path. There had to have been a whole host of people up there getting in on this experience: the ambulance drivers, the doctors and therapists, and my dearest friend, who is a physical therapist for children.

I believe we were all there, agreeing to our roles in this play. When I sit with those beliefs and simply breathe, I feel closer to acceptance and peace.

There is nothing to be done to reclaim the past. There is no way to erase what has been done. I need to work on loosening my grip on the Jessica-That-Was so I can fully embrace the Jessica-That-Is. She is changed, but she is every bit as amazing, pure, and beautiful as she was pre-accident. She proves this every single day.

As the years progress, she may not be the "fine" I believed her to be when I lay in the dirt beside her, hearing the voices of my Angels tell me so, but she will be her own version of fine. I offer up my Gratitude to The Universe for her Light, which shines bright enough to keep my darkness at bay.

For those days when I am so filled with anger and sadness, the Light and Joy can overwhelm. If I let them.

As I said on the day of the accident…when, unbeknownst to

me, the accident was happening… "I need to stop making such a damn big deal about things. Life is good. I need to let it be."

Even then.

Even now.

Just gotta let it be.

EPILOGUE

April 29, 2014

Four years post-accident, and we never had our Hollywood moment.

Jessica continues to progress and get stronger every day, and I am working to erase the words "her recovery" from my vernacular. *Recovery* means the act or process of recovering, especially from sickness, shock, or setback. *Or a restoration to a former or better condition.* Or the regaining of something lost.

I have lost the ability to believe in Jessica's "recovery." The psychic's prediction haunts me every day, as I continue to grieve for the Jessica-That-Was and work to accept and love the Jessica-That-Is.

I grieve for dreams of school dances and graduation walks, first kisses, driving lessons, college campus tours, and watching Jesse walk Jessica down the wedding aisle. I am grieving the loss of a life filled with adventure, trips abroad, and new experiences for our entire family to share.

While there is sorrow in this ever-present grief and the hole that has never healed, the beauty in the balance of The Universe allows me the joys, as well.

The joy of loving the Jessica-That-Is.

The Jessica-That-Is never lost her determination, her Spirit, the inner light of her soul shining through the darkness to save us all. She is bright and funny, full of laughter and joy.

From the moment she gets up in the morning, taking pride in putting together her own breakfast and getting ready for school without help, to the moment she lies down at night, trying to say "good night" and "I love you" clearly, Jessica works harder than any person I know.

Not only does she deal with the day-to-day activities of school and maneuver through both new and old friendships, but she continues to fight, every day, to regain everything we all take for granted.

She is not yet walking independently, and her speech is still not understandable 100 percent of the time, but both are getting stronger and easier with each passing day.

No longer does she want to go on an African safari or visit the Museum of Natural History in New York. She is content to stay home, playing UNO and Hedbanz with her sisters and working on her speech by singing along to the Frozen soundtrack, Taylor Swift, Garth Brooks, and Lady Gaga.

She is back in school full time, maintaining a 3.25 GPA in mainstream classes in the sixth grade.

One of the most important aspects of this journey is that, despite Jessica's claim of having a "terrible memory," she has retained much of it. She remembers how to read and do math, and she continues to love everything that made her happy prior to her debilitating accident. She is still passionate about music and loves to dance, and she remains a fan of Harry Potter, Percy Jackson and, of course, Collin Joseph. She cherishes visits with her family, laughs constantly at her dad's deadpan sense of humor, and, thankfully, still wants to be with me more than anywhere else.

Four years later, and I can't really do Jessica's progress or her recovery justice. How many ways can you describe a miracle? How many ways can you explain the defiance of deathly odds? Being spectacular, inspirational, and amazing?

I cannot express the depth of her humor and the quality of her laughter. The reasons for or the pain behind her tears. If she knows you, she will show you. In her own way and in her own time.

We are all in this boat on the sea with her. Sometimes we bob along, relaxing in the sun and ocean spray; sometimes we have to hang on, hoping not to capsize. We can help Jessica navigate the best we can, but she is the one in control. Gently, we row.

I no longer yearn to know what the future holds. I try to live in The Unknown, floating along, waiting to see where life takes us next.

Jessica is alive. Whatever will be, will be beautiful and miraculous by default.

There are far, far better things ahead than any we leave behind.
C. S. Lewis

ACKNOWLEDGEMENTS

Right up until Jessica's accident, I was the type of person who looked at the parents of children with special needs and said in admiration, "I don't know how you do it."

Or I would state with certainty, "I could never do it."

I'd like to think I actually tried to imagine how it would be if one of my children were "different," "handicapped," "differently abled," or "broken," but I don't think my thoughts went beyond admiring others for their strength and courage and offering up my Gratitude to The Universe for my children being healthy, strong, and able-bodied.

Had I sat down and truly tried to see things from a special-needs parent's perspective, I would have realized that it isn't just strength and courage that drives them but, more importantly, the love they have for their children. Viewed from that perspective, it is easy to see how they do what they do. How I now do what I do.

It is that inexplicable something in all of us. It is more than just keeping going when all you want to do is lie down and quit. It is stopping the moving bullet, outrunning the locomotive, defying gravity, and yes, moving the Earth.

What wouldn't we do for our children?

Thank you to everyone who believes I am doing this amazing thing. You would do the exact same thing, and I would be right there with you, cheering you on and pulling you forward, as you did for me.

For holding my heart in your heart, thank you to Kari Shipman, Libby Sullivan, Amanda Thronburg, Kelly Elliston, Jeff and Nicole Look, and Kathy Handley.

Thank you also:

...to Kathy Handley for inspiring and, really, providing 90 percent of the language in the book's prologue.

...to Amelia Jade, Collin Joseph, and Wendy Rose for making Jessica smile against all odds.

...to Melissa Reali, "Becky Masters," and Hannah Shipman for inspiring Jessica early on when the doctors doubted her ability to recover.

...to Lance Tressler for saving us from The Pit of Despair.

For the Love, Light, Energy, and Prayers that carried us along, I thank the Lavine Family Tree, the Gribbens Family Tree, Barb Jacobs and Family, the Tricks Dance Company 2006–2010 Families, the Dance Moms and Bench Time, Shannon and Mallory Jones, Cyndi Shreve and Jessica's Posse, our Brighton Family, our MyFolsom Family, Brian and Kim Johnson and Strings of Folsom, Cupcake Craving, the Folsom Telegraph, SacDJ, the Monday Night Supper Club, the kids of Blanche Sprentz Elementary School, the Oregon Contingent, Ms. Schabinger and Ms. Rymzsa, Momma and The Sisters (Julie Rapoza, Tricia Garcia, Dayna Garibay, and Christy Beville), and all of The Usual Suspects.

Thank you to the celebrities who touched our lives: Sara Bareilles for treating Jessica so sweetly at your Cafeteria 15L show and Marko Germar for dedicating your solo at the San Jose show for the 2011 *So You Think You Can Dance* tour to Jessica. To those singer-songwriters who have graciously permitted the use of their lyrics: Joni Mitchell and team for the use of the song "River," Fred Small for the use of the song "Everything Possible," and Sara Bareilles and team for the use of the songs "Gravity" and "Uncharted." To all the artists whose work inspired bits 'n pieces of this book, thank you for putting your gifts out into the world.

To my book team: Frances Kuffel – Thank you for doing the grunt work early on; Linda Stirling – you *are* the blessing; Diane Papadakis – for my amazing cover; Sandra Williams – for the flawless interior design; Sandi Corbitt-Sears – Thank you for helping to elevate my book to a level I didn't know it could reach; and Bruce McAllister – You *are* my loop; thank you for guiding me to the correct path and for speaking to the soul of my writing.

To all past and present members of the *Guide Her Home* Focus Group: Thank you for your reading, feedback, encouragement, and support. Special thanks for longevity to Kari Shipman, Kelly Elliston, Deb Boogaard, and Barb Jacobs.

Thanks to the Unitarian Universalist Church of Vancouver's Writer's Reading Group, the SW WA/OR Write to Publish Writing Group, and the Foothill Free Two Writing Group.

Thank you,

. . . to David Hammer, MA, MFT, and Debra Belshee-Storlie, Ph.D., for your compassion and understanding and for helping me tame my demons and believe in and trust myself.

. . . to the Children's Miracle Network, The Wolf 101.9, and all the radio stations nationwide for the work you do to support Children's Miracle Network hospitals, including UC Davis Children's Hospital.

. . . to the top contributors to my Night of Writing Dangerously: Lynne and Jud Clark and The Pekarek Family.

. . . to our "Your Name In Lights" (and beyond) IndieGoGo contributors: Laurie Andreoni; Lorena Angell; Deb Boogaard; Brenda Bridges-Cruz; Patrick Cleary; The Elliston Family; Nathan Gilbert; Rasee Govindani; Lisa Jones; Angela Juline; Jody Koch; Harry and Julie Lavine; Edward and Cathy Lehman; Jeff, Nicole, and Aidan Look; Debra Paschke; Ayiiia Pasterski; Melissa Reali; Kristin Rost; Kari Shipman; Kate Smith; Kimith So; Teresa Teachout; Marjorie Wilkison; and Jim Williams. Thank you to everyone who gave time, money, and energy to both campaigns.

Highest Love and Deepest Gratitude to all of the medical professionals who touched our daughter's life: South Placer Fire, Sutter Roseville Medical Center, UC Davis Children's Hospital, UC Davis Outpatient Therapy, and Legacy Health Children's Pediatric

Rehabilitation. Special thanks to Dr. Bosco, Dr. Chehrazi, Dr. Manhart, Dr. Davidson, Dr. Gerritz, Joan Holmes-Asamoah, Laurie Brown, Faye Diskin, and Nicole Mistretta.

To my Peanut Butter & Jelly: I could fill a thousand books with the many ways I am so very honored to be your mother. Jocelyn, this part is to you: Thank you for spinning through our lives, tossing out light and brightening everything you touch. I love you, Jocaruby. To the Jessica-That-Was, the Jessica-That-Is, and the Jessica-That-Will-Be: You are my very favorite Jessica. I love you the Bestica.

To Jesse: When I wrote my vows to you all those years ago, thanking you for allowing me to be weak, I never knew you would have to come through to this extent. Thank you for finding me in yet another life and being such an amazing father to our girls. As long as we're together, we can get through anything. Thank you for our Fairytale Life. I love you.

To Joy Drake and Kathy Taylor: Thank you for *The Transformation Game* and the amazing gift of the Angels.

And finally, to my Angels, Spirit, our Higher Selves, The Universe, God, Ra, Source, Creator, Maker, Buddah, Allah . . . To all that is Holy: Gratitude Rising. Thank you for hearing the meditations, prayers, chants, manifestations, and dances around the campfires shaking tambourines.

Thank you, even more, for answering them.

Blessed Be.

ABOUT THE AUTHOR

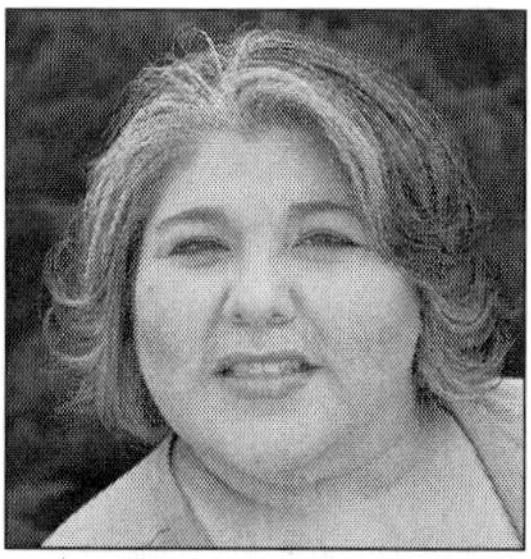

Photo by Jennifer Ross

Jolene Lavine is the married mom of two wonderful daughters, Jessica and Jocelyn. She believes in signs, following your gut instincts, supporting the underdog, and believing in the power of your dreams. She is a blissful Pacific Northwest resident who searches for the simple pleasures in life with her family and champions the beauty that can be found in the balance of The Universe.

When she is not laughing with and smooching her husband and kids, she spends her time writing, being crafty, singing along with Sara Bareilles at the top of her lungs, taking long LUSH baths and working quotes from *The Office* into every possible conversation.

Lovingly supported by her husband, Jesse, she is *finally* pursuing a career in writing.

Find her online: www.jolenelavine.com
www.facebook.com/jolenelavineauthor
www.facebook.com/guideherhome

14346148R00177

Made in the USA
San Bernardino, CA
23 August 2014